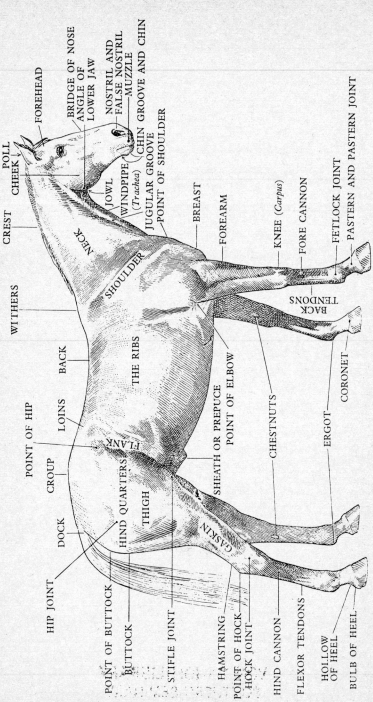

FOREHEAD
BRIDGE OF NOSE
ANGLE OF LOWER JAW
NOSTRIL AND FALSE NOSTRIL
MUZZLE
CHIN GROOVE AND CHIN
POINT OF SHOULDER
JUGULAR GROOVE
WINDPIPE (Trachea)
JOWL
CHEEK
POLL
CREST
NECK
WITHERS
SHOULDER
BACK
THE RIBS
LOINS
POINT OF HIP
CROUP
FLANK
DOCK
HIND QUARTERS
THIGH
HIP JOINT
POINT OF BUTTOCK
BUTTOCK
GASKIN
STIFLE JOINT
HAMSTRING
POINT OF HOCK
HOCK JOINT
HIND CANNON
FLEXOR TENDONS
HOLLOW OF HEEL
BULB OF HEEL
ERGOT
CORONET
CHESTNUTS
SHEATH OR PREPUCE
POINT OF ELBOW
BREAST
FOREARM
KNEE (Carpus)
FORE CANNON
BACK TENDONS
FETLOCK JOINT
PASTERN AND PASTERN JOINT

Fig. 1   The Points of the Horse.

(After Miller and Robertson)

Agricultural and Livestock Series

HORSE DISEASES

H. G. BELSCHNER, E.D., D.V.Sc., H.D.A., F.A.C.V.Sc.

Formerly Assistant Director of Veterinary Services,
First Cavalry Division, Australian Military Forces
—Eastern Command; Chief, Division of Animal Industry,
Department of Agriculture, New South Wales
and Senior Lecturer in Animal Management,
University of Sydney.

ANGUS AND ROBERTSON • PUBLISHERS

First published in 1969 by

ANGUS AND ROBERTSON (PUBLISHERS) PTY LTD
102 Glover Street, Cremorne, Sydney
2 Fisher Street, London
159 Boon Keng Road, Singapore
P.O. Box 1072, Makati MCC, Rizal, Philippines
115 Rosslyn Street, West Melbourne
222 East Terrace, Adelaide
1 Little Street, Fortitude Valley, Brisbane

Second Edition (Revised) 1974

© Belschner Literary (Holdings) Limited 1969

Card number and ISBN 0 207 12930 4

PRINTED IN AUSTRALIA BY JOHN SANDS PTY LTD
HALSTEAD PRESS DIVISION

PREFACE

THE PURPOSE of this book is to describe briefly, in simple language, the more common diseases and injuries to which the horse is prone. The more important ones are dealt with in greater detail.

The book is written primarily for the average horse-owner, such as the farmer, grazier, pony club member and so on, with the object of providing up-to-date knowledge on those diseases and injuries of the horse with which they are more likely to come in contact. It is appreciated that many horse-owners have little knowledge of the anatomy and physiology of the horse and therefore scientific names have been kept to an absolute minimum and common names and horse terms have been used. There are many fanciful names given to certain disease conditions of the horse, such as "thoroughpin", which inaptly describes the condition. They have been handed down by farriers and others and the names are still accepted.

The treatments given are in the main along first-aid lines, having in mind what the average horse-owner might accomplish with available facilities and readily accessible drugs, when professional assistance is not available. Good nursing is stressed.

With the increasing numbers of University qualified veterinary surgeons available throughout the country, horse-owners are able to obtain expert advice and treatment for sick and injured animals, and it is recommended that such assistance should be obtained wherever possible.

Veterinarians have at their disposal a great number of valuable ethical drugs which are not available to the horse-owner, and, furthermore, have the necessary equipment and instruments so often essential for effective treatment.

Antibiotic and sulphonamide drugs now play a very important part in the treatment of many diseases and, although some of these drugs are available to the general public, they are of little value unless carefully selected according to the type of disease and properly administered at adequate dose rates.

No attempt has been made to describe every disease which affects horses nor to discuss in detail certain obscure lamenesses which, in any case, would come within the province of a veterinarian. I have been content, in order to keep the book at a reasonable size, to deal with the main disease conditions and those likely to be seen and recognized, perhaps with the aid of this text, by the horse-owner. The diseases have been listed in alphabetical order for quick reference.

Although *Horse Diseases* has been written primarily for the horse-owner, it is suggested that it will be found useful as a text book in Agricultural Colleges and other establishments where elementary veterinary science or animal health is taught as part of the curriculum.

In the preparation of this book certain standard reference books and articles in scientific journals have been consulted, a list of which is given with due acknowledgement.

I wish to acknowledge the permission granted by the New South Wales Department of Agriculture, the United States Department of Agriculture and the Veterinary Department of the War Office, London, to quote from various publications and to reproduce certain plates and figures.

I am indebted to the authors and publishers of various books for permission to reproduce certain plates and figures to illustrate some sections of the book.

I also gratefully acknowledge the generous assistance given me by Mr. R. H. Falk, B.V.Sc., in checking the typescript and in making valuable suggestions and Miss Virginia Osborne, B.V.Sc., M.A.C.V.Sc., for assistance with colours and markings of horses.

Miranda   H.G.B.

New South Wales
Australia

CONTENTS

Abortion 1
Abscess 2
Anaemia 3
Anthrax 4
Appetite—"Depraved" 5
Azoturia 5

Back and Loins 7
Big Head (Osteomalacia) 8
Bladder, Eversion of 8
Bladder, Inflammation of (Cystitis) 9
Bladder, Retention of Urine 10
Bleeding From Veins 11
Bleeding From Nose (Epistaxis) 12
Blistering 13
Blood Poisoning 13
Bone—Inflammation of 14
Bots 15
Botryomycosis 20
Botulism (Forage Poisoning) 20
Bowels—Inflammation (Enteritis) 22
Brain—Inflammation and Diseases of 24
Bran Mash—Preparation of 24
Broken Wind (Pulmonary Emphysema) 24
Bronchitis 26
Brushing 26
Burns 27

Calculi 29
Cancer 29
Canker 30
Capped Elbow 31
Capped Hock 32
Cataract 34
Catarrh (Acute Nasal) ("Colds") 34
Choking 35
Colic 36
Colours and Markings 250
Corns 45
Cracked Heels 46
Crib-Biting and Wind-Sucking 47
Curb 49

Dentition and Ageing 50
Destruction of a Horse 67
Diarrhoea 67
Diarrhoea in Foals 68
Dislocations 69
Displacement of The Patella (Stifle Slip) 70
Drenching Horses ·72

Eczema 73
Emphysema 74
Encephalomyelitis—Viral 75
Equine Infectious Anaemia (Swamp Fever) 76
Eye—Foreign Bodies in 79
Eye—Conjunctivitis 79
Eye—Keratitis 81
Eye—Habronemic Conjunctivitis 82
Eye—Periodic Ophthalmia 83
Eye—"Dermoid Cysts" 84
Eyelids—Entropion 84

False Quarter 85
Fistula 86
Fistulous Withers and Poll Evil 86
Flies 89
Foal—Rearing of Orphan 91
Founder—Laminitis 92
Fractures 95
Frog—Diseases of 96

Gastro-Enteritis 97
Girth Galls 98
Grease—Greasy Heel 99

Heart Diseases 100
Heatstroke—Heat Exhaustion—Sunstroke 100
Hernia (Rupture) 101
Hock—Diseases of 103
Hoof—Diseases of 104

Indigestion (Dyspepsia) 106
"Influenza"—Equine 107
Infectious Equine Bronchitis 108

Jaundice (Icterus) 109
Joint-Ill (Navel Ill) 109

Knees, Broken   111
Kidneys—Inflammation of (Nephritis)   112
Kimberley or Walkabout Disease   114

Lameness   115
Lampas (Palatitis)   117
Laryngitis   118
Leg Mange ("Itchy Heel")   119
Lice   120
Lymphangitis (Sporadic)   123

Mange   125
Mastitis (Inflammation of the Udder)   125
Melanoma   126
Metritis (Inflammation of the Uterus)   126
Myositis—Acute (Tying-up or Cording-up)   127

Navicular Disease   128
Nettle Rash (Urticaria, Hives)   130
Nursing a Sick Horse   131

Paralysis   132
Parasites—Internal   133
Parturition   143
Pervious Urachus ("Leaking Navel")   151
Periostitis   151
Peritonitis   152
Photosensitization (Trefoil Dermatitis)   153
Pleurisy   154
Pneumonia   156
Poisoning (Plant and Mineral)   157
Polyps   161
Pregnancy   162
Purpura Haemorrhagica   163

Queensland Itch   164
Quidding   166
Quittor   167

Retention of Afterbirth   167
Rig   169
Ringbone   169
Ringworm   171
Roaring and Whistling   174

Saddle Galls—Sore Backs   175
Salivary Calculi (Cheek Stones)   185

Sandcrack 185
Scirrhous Cord 188
Seedy Toe 189
Sesamoiditis 190
Shoeing 190
Shoeing Pricks 191
Shoulder Lameness 192
Sidebone 195
Sitfast 197
Sleepy Foal Disease (Shigellosis) 197
Sore Shins (Periostitis, Ostitis) 198
Spavin 199
Speedy-Cut 203
Splints 204
Sprung Hock 208
Staggers 208
Stomach—Rupture of 209
Strangles 210
Stringhalt 213
Superpurgation 216
Suppression of Urine 217

Teeth—Irregularities of Molars 218
Temperature, Pulse and Respiration 219
Tendons—Sprained 221
Tetanus 222
Thoroughpin 225
Thrush 227
Tongue—Inflammation of 229
Tuberculosis 229
Tumours 230
Twisted Bowel 231

Ulcer 232
Urinary Calculi ("Stone" or "Gravel") 233

Vaginitis 235

Warts 236
Watering 237
Weaving 237
Weed 238
Weights and Measures 238
Windgalls 242
Wounds 243

Appendix: Colours and Markings of Horses for
    Identification Purposes 250

ILLUSTRATIONS

LIST OF FIGURES

1	Points of the horse	*frontispiece*
2	Circulation of the Blood	11
3	Bot-fly larvae	16
4	Normal stomach of horse—lining membranes	17
5	Life history of botflies	19
6	Capped hock	33
7	Stomach of horse	37
8	Abdominal viscera of horse	40
9	Viscera of mare	41
10	Teeth of a crib-biter	47
11	Curb	49
12	Diagram of incisor tooth	55
13	Dentition and Ageing—Mouth at one week	56
14	Mouth at four to six weeks	56
15	Mouth at five to six months	56
16	Mouth at one year	56
17	Mouth at two years	57
18	Tables of lower incisors at two years	57
19	Mouth rising three years	57
20	Tables of lower incisors at rising three years	57
21	Mouth at three years past	58
22	Tables of lower incisors at three years past	58
23	Mouth rising four years	58
24	Tables of lower incisors at rising four years	58
25	Mouth at four years	59
26	Tables of lower incisors at four years	59
27	Mouth rising five years	59
28	Tables of lower incisors at rising five years	59
29	Mouth at five years	60
30	Tables of lower incisors at five years	60
31	Mouth at six years	61
32	Tables of lower incisors at six years	61
33	Mouth at seven years	62
34	Tables of lower incisors at seven years	62
35	Mouth at eight years	63
36	Tables of lower incisors at eight years	63
37	Mouth at nine years	64
38	Tables of lower incisors at nine years	64
39	Mouth at ten years	65
40	Tables of lower incisors at ten years	65
41	Mouth at eleven years	65
42	Tables of lower incisors at eleven years	65

43	Mouth at twelve years	66
44	Tables of lower incisors at twelve years	66
45	Eye of horse	81
46	Fistulous Wither	87
47	Poll Evil	89
48	Section of a foot with laminitis of 8 days standing	93
49	Section of a foot with laminitis of 14 days standing	93
50	Umbilical Hernia	102
51	Urinary organs of horse	113
52	Section of kidney of horse	114
53	Biting louse of horse	121
54	Sucking louse of horse	122
55	Life history of Red Worms	134
56	The Large Roundworm	136
57	Life history of Large Roundworm	137
58	Life history of Large Stomach Worms	140
59	Pinworms and eggs	142
60	Normal presentations of the foetus	144
61	Abnormal presentations of the foetus	147
62	Abnormal presentation—thigh and croup	148
63	Abnormal presentation—hind limb deviation	148
64	Abnormal presentation—transverse	149
65	Abnormal presentation—sterno-abdominal	149
66	Abnormal presentation—head turned on side	150
67	Abnormal presentation—head turned on back	150
68	Queensland Itch	165
69	Ringbone	170
70	Ringworm	172
71	The skeleton of the horse	177
72	Dorsal and lumbar regions of the horse	179
73	The muscles of the horse	181
74	Sandcracks	187
75	Anatomy and diseases of the foot	194
76	Sidebone	196
77	Bone spavin	200
78	Bog spavin	200
79	Bone spavin—lesions	201
80	Splint	205
81	Stringhalt	214
82	Skull of horse—molar teeth	218
83	Thoroughpin	226

COLOUR PLATES

Between pages 114 and 115

1 Splints
2 Ringbone
3 Anatomy of the foot
4 Anatomy of the foot

ABORTION

ABORTION is the premature expulsion of the foetus, or of the contents of the pregnant uterus (womb). If the foal is advanced enough to live, the act is referred to as premature parturition. Most twins are aborted before full term. Abortion can occur at any time between the first and tenth months of pregnancy. With very few exceptions, foals born one month before full term (11 months approximately) cannot live.

Causes

By far the most common cause of abortion is infection, either bacterial, fungal or viral. Many organisms are known to be responsible for causing abortion in mares, but the latest research has shown that two viruses of the upper respiratory tract known as *equine viral rhinopneumonitis* (EVR) and *equine viral arteritis* (EVA), are responsible for severe outbreaks of infective abortion in mares in the United States of America and elsewhere. This so-called "virus abortion" has been recorded in Australia, but as yet does not appear to have assumed great importance as a cause of abortion in mares in this country.

Non-specific abortions do occur sporadically, and abortion can also occur as a direct or indirect consequence of certain systemic diseases. Hormonal imbalance in the mare may occasionally result in abortion.

The diagnosis of the cause must be left to a veterinarian in collaboration with laboratory workers.

Symptoms

Abortions are frequently associated with metritis (inflammation of the uterus) and in this respect the symptoms are similar to Brucellosis in cattle. A sticky rust-coloured discharge may be noticed a few days before the act of abortion and this continues after the abortion has occurred. Early abortions may take place without any warning symptoms, and may not be seen. In such cases, the first indication that this event has taken place is that the mare comes in season again. With early abortions, the membranes are usually discharged with the foetus. When they occur in the later months of pregnancy, the placenta or portion thereof may be retained, to be followed by a severe metritis (inflammation of the uterus) with persistent discharge from the vulva. Other than by microscopical examination of smears from discharges, or by blood or other tests, it is not possible to say whether the abortion has been due to a specific infection. If abortions have occurred in a number of mares, suspicion would be aroused.

1

Treatment

Mares showing indications of having aborted, or of impending abortion, should be immediately isolated. The foetus, its membranes and any discharges should be burnt. Professional assistance should be obtained without delay, so that wide spectrum antibiotic and other forms of treatment can be carried out early. Antibiotics are not likely to have any effect against the viral infections, for which there is no specific treatment, but will be of value against secondary infections and against bacterial infections generally. The affected mare or mares will require good nursing, and the strictest sanitary measures should be practised. The mare should not be served again for a month or longer, and in no case until after all discharges from the vulva have ceased and the animal appears to be in normal health.

ABSCESS

AN ABSCESS is a localized collection of pus which may occur anywhere on the body and is sometimes deep seated. Internal abscesses also occur. A small superficial abscess is known as a pustule. Abscesses may be acute or chronic and should not be confused with haematomas, due to bruising and extravasation of blood. An acute abscess is a hot painful swelling which develops rapidly with formation of pus. The swelling gradually increases in size, comes to a head and bursts. A chronic abscess is one which takes a long time to develop, is frequently deep seated and seldom bursts unless near the surface. Examples of chronic abscesses are those seen in poll evil and fistulous withers. Deep seated abscesses occur not uncommonly in the shoulder, at the base of the neck and in the hind quarter.

Cause

Generalized infections, which occur in certain specific diseases such as strangles in the horse, or infection of some local injury by various types of bacteria are the causes of abscesses.

Symptoms

The first symptom of an acute external abscess is a hard swelling, gradually increasing in size. This swelling is usually hot and painful and, depending on its size, may be accompanied by a rise in temperature and interference with the function of the part. The abscess bulges or "points" at some particular spot and eventually bursts. Should this occur at a spot where good drainage can take place, the pus is evacuated, the pain ceases and the temperature drops. In some deep seated abscesses the pus may never reach the surface, although the skin over the area may be slightly swollen, painful and "pit" on pressure. In such cases absorption results and the abscess becomes encapsulated in fibrous tissue. There is always the danger, with such a chronic abscess, that a sinus or fistula will occur.

Internal abscesses which burst into an internal cavity may lead to septic infection and death, or prolonged ill-health of the animal.

Treatment

The treatment for an acute external abscess is to hasten its *ripening* by hot fomentations, the use of liniments and sometimes even by light blistering. If a blister is used, care should be taken to prevent it running by placing a ring of petroleum jelly around the area being blistered. When the abscess is soft, it should be opened at the lowest part with a sharp clean knife. After allowing the pus to drain, the cavity might be syringed out with some weak antiseptic solution, or a teaspoonful of salt to a pint of water. This may have to be repeated. It is necessary to keep the wound open until the cavity has drained properly. If all the pus has been evacuated the cavity rapidly heals. A chronic or deep seated abscess will require the use of antibiotics and the services of a veterinary surgeon.

AGE BY THE TEETH

See *Dentition and Ageing*

ANAEMIA

ANAEMIA is a term applied to a deficiency of red blood corpuscles, or haemoglobin, per unit volume of blood.

Cause

Anaemia is no longer considered as a primary disease, but as a symptom of some other disorder. We refer broadly to haemorrhagic anaemia which occurs after severe haemorrhage, or with chronic blood loss due to internal and external parasites, and to haemolytic anaemia which occurs in many infectious and non-infectious diseases.

Symptoms

Pallor of the visible mucous membranes of the eyes, nose and mouth, a rapid weak pulse, cold extremities and muscular weakness are the main manifestations of anaemia. Lesser degrees of anaemia may occur, particularly in the horse, when whiteness of the mucous membranes does not occur and other definite symptoms are not shown, but performance is affected. Such cases are commonly associated with red worm infection.

3

B

Treatment

It is essential that the primary cause of the anaemia be treated. Non-specific treatment includes blood transfusions in the case of severe haemorrhage, and in less severe cases the use of haematinic preparations which increase the haemoglobin content of the blood. Iron may be given by mouth in the form of syrup of phosphate of iron, 1 tablespoonful twice daily. Vitamin B_{12} is often used as a non-specific treatment for anaemia. Nutritious food, plenty of green-stuff and well-regulated exercise are indicated.

ANTHRAX

ANTHRAX is an acute infectious disease of a septicaemic nature which may affect any animal. The disease is of world-wide distribution and is more commonly seen in herbivorous animals including the horse. Man is also susceptible and may contract the disease at a post-mortem examination.

Cause

The disease is caused by a specific organism, *Bacillus anthracis*, gaining entrance to the body.

Symptoms

The initial symptoms are high fever, general depression, and frequently, especially in the horse, severe pains resembling those of colic or acute enteritis. Later, swellings may occur on different parts of the body including the neck, throat, chest, along the abdomen and on the legs. There may be a blood-stained discharge from the nose and anus, but usually this is not shown until after death. Horses commonly exhibit a longer course of the disease than other animals, but death usually occurs in one or two days.

Treatment

There is no treatment. If the disease is suspected it should be reported immediately to the nearest veterinary inspector or other authority.

The disease is confirmed by microscopic examination of a blood smear from the affected animal. The sick horse should be placed in isolation and fowls and dogs kept away. If the animal dies before the authorities arrive, no attempt should be made to carry out a post-mortem examination, as it is very dangerous to open the carcase. A tarpaulin or bags should be thrown over the carcase to cover it and all discharges completely. Subsequently the carcase should be burnt or deeply buried and covered with a thick layer of unslaked lime. The authorities will advise concerning any disinfection of premises which may be necessary.

APPETITE—"DEPRAVED"

SOMETIMES a horse will eat earth, cinders, stones, plastic, bark of trees, dung and other rubbish. This is referred to as "pica", which means a depraved appetite for unnatural food, and varies from licking to actual eating.

Bark-eating is a fairly common habit amongst horses in certain districts, and is a cause of some concern to owners. The horses strip off the bark sometimes to the extent of ring-barking the tree. No ill effects may result if the bark is not eaten to excess, but it can cause serious digestive upsets and obstruction of the bowels, as can the ingestion of other foreign matter.

Causes

The cause is usually some mineral deficiency, such as calcium (lime), or phosphate, but it is not always easy to determine what mineral deficiency exists. In many cases it appears that the trouble is due to a calcium-phosphorus imbalance, especially when horses are fed mainly on a straight cereal chaff-oats-bran ration. It sometimes occurs when salt is not fed in the ration or made available as rock-salt. Worm infection, protein deficiency, or any form of stomach or bowel irritation, can be responsible. Boredom may be a cause, if animals are closely confined.

Prevention

Quite often the habit of bark-eating in particular can be prevented by feeding liberal amounts of good-quality lucerne chaff or lucerne hay, which is a fodder rich in both protein and calcium. An alternative way of supplying lime, other than through lucerne, is to add $1\frac{1}{2}$ oz. of finely ground limestone to the daily ration, well mixed in the feed. 1 oz. of salt should also be added to the daily ration, or rock-salt made available. Routine treatments for the control of stomach bots and intestinal worms may be required.

AZOTURIA

THIS disease, the modern name of which is *paralytic myoglobinuria* and which is also referred to as *haemoglobinuria* and "red water" or "black water", was once a common and serious disease in working draught horses. It is not now so commonly seen, but does occur in light horses, though usually in a mild form. The disease is characterized by paralysis of certain muscles, which appears during exercise

5

following a short period of idleness on a full working diet, and thus one common name for the disease is "Monday morning sickness". The term azoturia, meaning nitrogen in the urine, was found to be a misnomer, but use of the name has become traditional.

In racing stables the term "tied up" or "cording up" is used to describe what appears to be a mild form of azoturia, but may be a separate disease. (See *Myositis*)

Cause

The exact cause of the disease is not known but the conditions under which it occurs are well defined, as referred to above. It has been suggested that when horses accustomed to regular work are allowed to rest for several days on full rations, some derangement in the process of conversion of carbohydrates in tissues occurs with the accumulation of lactic acid in the tissues and blood. This produces a myopathy or muscle disease. When the horse works after being spelled, the muscle fibres break down and muscle pigment is liberated, passes into the blood and is excreted by the kidneys. It is not a kidney disease, although in some cases the kidneys may subsequently be involved.

A new approach to the study of the cause of the disease has followed the recent discovery of the roles of selenium and vitamin E in other forms of muscle disease and in metabolism.

Symptoms

The main symptoms of this disease are the suddenness of the attack; lameness usually in a hind limb; muscle trembling; profuse sweating; panting; crouching; dark coloured urine; paralysis; spasms and collapse.

Treatment

Veterinary attention as soon as possible is very desirable. Should there be delay in obtaining professional assistance, the horse should be kept as quiet as possible and every effort made to keep it standing. A purgative drench, such as 1 to 2 quarts of liquid paraffin or a pint of raw linseed oil, should be carefully administered. The horse might also be "back-raked", and an enema given. If the animal goes down, it should be made as comfortable as possible with a bedding of thick straw and turned over every few hours to prevent bedsores. If the horse is out in the open, a temporary shelter should be erected, and a rug thrown over the animal. No attempt should be made to walk the horse any distance. If it is desired to move it, this should be done by low-level trailer. Arrangements should be made for watering the animal, and green feed and bran mashes included in a light laxative diet. No grain should be fed. The daily administration of sodium bicarbonate (baking soda), 3 to 4 oz. daily in the feed or as a drench in water, is recommended. Repeated hot fomentations and massage of affected muscles are of value. Good nursing is essential.

Modern treatment includes intramuscular injections of thiamine hydrochloride, the administration of antihistamines and vitamin E and the use of tranquillizers. If the urine is retained, it will need to be drawn off with a catheter by a veterinary surgeon.

BACK AND LOINS

SPRAINS and injury to the muscles of the back and those of the loins, and changes in the spinal column occur from time to time and are often responsible for obscure lameness.

Cause

Violent efforts, powerful muscular strains, jumping, slipping and falling are some of the causes of sprains and injury in this region. Ankylosis (union) of the vertebrae following some injury such as a bad fall, injury to the back resulting in the formation of fibrous tissue in the muscles, and even injury to the spinal cord, are other less common causes.

Symptoms

A series of symptoms are shown when the back and loins are injured and it is frequently difficult to determine just where the trouble is. The common symptoms are partial paralysis of the hind limbs; the animal is unable to back or turn properly; pain is shown on pressure over the back and loins; the back droops under weight and there may be partial or complete inability to lift the tail. In lying down the horse seems to suffer much discomfort and often groans as it goes down. When compelled to rise, it does so with difficulty and seldom suceeds without repeated efforts.

The condition is often referred to as "jinked-back".

Treatment

The first and most important treatment is rest. The horse should be placed in a sling in a narrow stall. Hot compresses, cold douches, stimulating liniments, massage and diathermy (electrical stimulation) may be beneficial. The prognosis depends on the cause, but in any case a long rest is generally necessary and the patient may not make a complete recovery.

If a horse falls at a hurdle or, as a result of some other injury is unable to support itself behind, even when lifted up on to its feet, it may be concluded that the back has been broken, and it should be destroyed.

BARK-EATING

See *Appetite—"Depraved"*

BIG HEAD (Osteomalacia)

OSTEOMALACIA is a general term used to describe softening of the bones and is sometimes incorrectly referred to as *adult rickets*. In cattle more particularly, the bones of affected animals become swollen, soft and spongy and are easily broken. In horses the bones of the skull are often involved and the head shows a grossly swollen appearance, hence the common name "big head". It occurs chiefly in mature animals.

Cause

The cause of the disease is not fully understood, but it appears to be associated with either a deficient intake or absorption of calcium or phosphorus, or to increased excretion of either of these elements, or to a calcium-phosphorus imbalance. A deficiency of vitamin D or trace elements may contribute to the condition.

Symptoms

Swelling of bones of the face, generally midway between eyes and nose and under the surface of the jaw. There is usually no pain, but the teeth may be loosened.

Treatment

Unless the specific dietary deficiencies can be determined it is impossible to treat the animal intelligently. Change of feed and locality sometimes arrests the condition. Lucerne hay or lucerne chaff should be added to the ration, or 1½ oz. of finely-ground limestone supplied daily in the feed.

BIRDSVILLE DISEASE

See under *Kimberley or Walkabout Disease*

BLADDER, EVERSION OF

EVERSION of the bladder may occur before or during foaling. It is much more common in mares than in the cow or sow and is associated with violent parturition. The bladder turns inside out through the channel of the urethra and protrudes through the lips of the vulva.

Symptoms

Straining, and the appearance of a red pear-shaped mass hanging from the floor of the vulva and protruding between the lips. The openings of the two ureters into the bladder drip urine.

Treatment

The replacement of the everted organ usually requires the service of a veterinarian. If professional assistance is not available, cleanse the protruding organ with weak antiseptic solution or simply wash with warm water and soap; massage the organ carefully and then with clean soapy hands gently, firmly and continuously press in and down until the organ slips into place. If this is found to be impossible owing to swelling, wind a strip of two-inch bandage tightly around the protruding organ to express the blood and diminish its bulk, and gradually unwind the bandage as the bladder is pushed back. Should the mare be straining violently, a sedative, such as 1 oz. of chloral hydrate in a quart of water, should be given as a drench. Subsequent treatment consists of irrigating the bladder with sterile normal saline solution and antibiotics, and the injection of antibiotics intramuscularly or subcutaneously to control infection.

BLADDER, INFLAMMATION OF (Cystitis)

INFLAMMATION of the bladder is mostly caused by bacterial infection, but it may also be caused by the excretion of irritant substances in the urine following overdosing with turpentine, saltpetre and other drugs, or the application of blistering ointments containing cantharides or mercury compounds over an extensive area of the skin. The presence of large or irregular shaped calculi ("stones") in the bladder not uncommonly causes inflammation of the wall of the bladder. The use of an unclean catheter is a means of conveying bacteria into the bladder. In other cases bacteria gain entrance to the bladder through the ureters, from a diseased kidney, and in mares from the genital passages through the short urethra. Sudden exposure of a sweating and tired horse to cold and wet conditions can be a cause, as can the presence of certain plants in the fodder. Inflammation of the bladder may also occur in the course of certain specific diseases.

Symptoms

The symptoms are repeated efforts to urinate and slight or severe colicky pains. The urine, which is passed in small quantities, may be clear or red or more commonly flocculent. The urine comes in spurts and is accompanied by signs of pain, which persists after the discharge, as shown by continued straining, groaning, and sometimes by movement of the feet and tail. The animal may kick at the abdomen, look around at the flank and lie down and rise frequently. When the condition is due to bacterial infection there is commonly a rise in temperature and accelerated pulse and respirations. If due to calculi, these may often be felt by palpation of the bladder with an oiled hand passed into the rectum, or in the case of a mare, with a finger passed through the urethral opening on the floor of the vagina.

Some of the above symptoms are similar to those seen in mild cases of spasmodic colic, from which the condition must be differentiated.

Treatment

First remove any suspected cause if possible. If there is evidence that the trouble is associated with blistering, the blistered part should be well washed with soap and water. If the urine has been retained and decomposed, it should be completely evacuated through a catheter and the bladder irrigated with a saturated solution of boric acid or other mild antiseptic solution, but this is a matter for a veterinarian. Certain drugs classed as urinary antiseptics may be given by the mouth or injected hypodermically or may be used in irrigating the bladder. Hot fomentations over the loins and in the perineum are sometimes of advantage. Luke-warm water injections should also be given by the rectum, and a drench of 8 oz. of Epsom salts in $1\frac{1}{2}$ pt of water should be administered. The diet should be light and should include linseed mashes, oatmeal gruels, hay tea or barley water.

BLADDER—RETENTION OF URINE

SPASM of the bladder and inability to pass urine can occur following hard and continuous riding or driving without the horse having an opportunity to pass urine. It may occur when the horse is exposed to cold rainstorms over a prolonged period, or becomes chilled from cold winds or draughts when sweating and fatigued. The condition sometimes accompanies severe impaction of the bowels (*impaction colic*) and other diseases. It may also be due to the presence of a "stone" in the urethra.

Symptoms

Frequent stretching and straining to urinate with no result or with only a slight dribble, is the main symptom shown. Later, evidence of pain is indicated by the horse kicking at the belly, moving uneasily, shaking the tail, arching the back, looking around at the flank and showing general signs of uneasiness. If an oiled hand is passed into the rectum, the distended bladder may be felt beneath and the horse will cringe when it is pressed. Examination per rectum may also reveal impaction of the bowel.

Treatment

The most effective treatment for retention of urine due to prolapse of the bladder is to pass a well-oiled horse catheter. This is a technical procedure which, except in an emergency, should be entrusted only to a veterinarian. In the mare, the neck of the bladder may be dilated by inserting two oiled fingers through the vagina into the short urethra. In the horse, the oiled hand introduced into the rectum can be pressed down on the bladder, sometimes with good effect. A warm water enema and hot fomentations over the loins are also of value. If a horse is placed in a stable, clean litter placed beneath the belly, and the animal left alone, it may urinate after a short rest.

BLEEDING FROM VEINS

BLEEDING or venesection was at one time employed in the treatment of a great many diseases of horses, and was also adopted in human medicine. It is now seldom carried out although there are occasions, such as in the case of high blood pressure, congestion of the lungs or acute laminitis (founder), when its use might be justified. The blood-

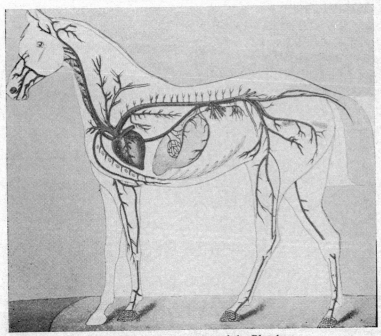

Fig. 2 The Circulation of the Blood.
(After Schwarz and Fleming)

letting is usually done from the jugular vein, having regard to the state of the pulse, by distending the vein with pressure from the fingers or the use of a cord around the neck, and withdrawing the blood with a bleeding needle. The blood should escape rapidly and a careful watch kept on the pulse. It is preferable for bleeding to be undertaken by a veterinary surgeon. Blood is also sometimes collected from the jugular vein for diagnostic purposes.

Accidental bleeding from veins as a result of injury is usually not serious. Venous blood is darker in colour than arterial blood, flows freely from the vessels and does not spurt out in a jerky stream. The best means of stopping bleeding is by pressure which may be carried out by tight bandaging over a pad of lint or folded clean cloth. Bleeding stops because the blood clots in the mouths of the wounded vessels. If a large vein has been cut and can be seen, it should be picked up with sterilized forceps and tied with sterilized catgut or cotton.

See also under *Wounds*

BLEEDING FROM NOSE (Epistaxis)

NOSE bleeding occurs during the course of certain diseases and may be a symptom of polypus or tumour in the nose. It can, however, occur independently of disease conditions and be due to violent exertions such as racing, injuries to the head or violent sneezing, which cause a rupture of small blood vessels in the nose. It not uncommonly occurs following inexpert use of a stomach tube.

Symptoms

In simple nose bleed the bleeding is usually from one nostril only and is not serious. The blood escapes in drops, seldom in a stream, and is not frothy as when the haemorrhage is from the lungs, when it is always from both nostrils.

Treatment

The treatment for simple bleeding from the nose consists of bathing the head with cold water. If the bleeding still continues an ice-pack to the head, ice-water over the face and plugging the nostril with cotton wool should be tried. It is advisable to tie a piece of string to the cotton wool plug so that it can safely be withdrawn after a few hours. The animal must be rested. If the bleeding is profuse and persistent, the services of a veterinarian should be obtained without delay.

BLISTERING

BLISTERS are applied directly to the skin for counter-irritation externally. Various medicinal substances are used for the purpose in the form of liquids and ointments. They vary from mild applications of mustard paste and liniments containing ammonia and oil of turpentine, to the more severe blistering ointments which contain cantharides, red iodide of mercury (red precipitate ointment), and other materials.

The object of counter-irritation is to set up a new inflammatory process in an area, which stimulates it to continue the work of healing and repair. It also promotes the absorption of adjacent enlargements. Care should be taken not to blister too severely.

Application of a Blister

The area to be blistered should be clipped closely, and then a ring of petroleum jelly placed around it to prevent the blister from running. An ointment blister is usually rubbed briskly into the skin for 5 to 10 minutes. Some liquid blisters are applied with a brush and not rubbed in. The horse should be tied up for 24 hours with two side-reins to prevent biting the blistered part. The tail should be secured if the blistered part is within its reach. A blistered horse must be kept under close observation to prevent self-mutilation. Blisters should not be applied during very hot weather.

It is difficult to stop the action of a blister which has proved to be too severe. The area can be washed with warm water and soap and then some cooling astringent lotion applied.

BLOOD POISONING (Septicaemia— Gas Gangrene—Pyaemia)

BY THE popular term "blood poisoning" is meant a general infection of the blood-stream by organisms of various types. This may be of a specific nature such as in the case of anthrax, or may be the result of infection of wounds by organisms of the "gas gangrene group" which thrive in the absence of air, or other organisms which need air for best growth. Further, pyogenic (pus-forming) organisms circulating in the blood usually cause abscess formation in various parts of the body. Mixed infections of various types of organisms commonly occur.

Causes

When not due to a specific infectious disease, septicaemia usually results from wound infection, especially punctured wounds in the feet of horses and elsewhere on the body; extensive wounds or inflamed areas; bone and joint injuries; difficult parturition, or following operations such as castration, extraction of teeth and bleeding.

Symptoms

All forms of septicaemia are serious. It is not uncommon for a horse to die suddenly, the only signs observed being a very high temperature and loss of appetite. In other cases there is shivering, fever, sweating, laboured respiration and heart action, and haemorrhages on the visible mucous membranes.

Treatment

Prompt antibiotic treatment and injections of antisera (where appropriate) by a veterinarian.

BONE—INFLAMMATION OF

PROBABLY bone diseases are responsible for more unfitness of horses than are any other type of ailments. The usefulness of large numbers of racehorses, trotters and other light horses is often temporarily or permanently lost through some bone affection, which may interfere with the movement of a joint. In addition, acute inflammation of the bone which commonly results from some external violence, such as a kick, often results in at least temporary unfitness and may lead to complications including exostosis (extra deposit of bone).

ACUTE INFLAMMATION

Bones are covered with a fibrous membrane known as the periosteum, except at the points of tendinous and ligamentous attachment and on the articular surfaces where cartilage is substituted. On those bones which are not deeply seated, as in the legs, the periosteum is easily injured by a blow and the result is very painful. Acute inflammation of bone may be divided into *periostitis* (inflammation of the periosteum), *osteitis* or *ostitis* (inflammation of the bone substance itself) and acute *osteomyelitis* (inflammation of the bone and central marrow cavity). These conditions may be progressive unless correctly treated.

Cause

Acute inflammation usually arises from external injuries which result from stumbling, falling, being kicked, striking hurdles and so on. It may arise from constitutional disturbance. Injury frequently involves some damage to ligament or tendon sheaths at points along their course, with inflammation spreading to the periosteum in the near vicinity. Bacterial contamination may aggravate the condition.

A condition known as "sore shins" affects the cannon bones of

14

young horses, especially thoroughbreds when their training has been too severe or they have been worked on very hard ground. This is ascribed to a periostitis.

Symptoms

Pain is usually evident when the affected part is handled and, if the trouble is in a limb bone, lameness results. The area is at first swollen and hot to the touch. Later the pain and heat are less but the thickening on the bone often remains for long periods. In severe cases where infection has occurred, there is a rise in temperature and the horse is dull and off its feed. Very mild cases of periostitis may show few symptoms and the condition is often overlooked until it is revealed by exostosis.

Treatment

Complete rest is essential. Hot fomentations, followed by the continuous application of cold water from a hose, and the use of cooling and soothing liniments, combined with rest, are usually sufficient to cut short mild attacks of acute inflammation of the bone. The earlier treatment is commenced, the more favourable is the prognosis. Iodine ointment is of value when the acute symptoms have subsided. More severe cases of ostitis and osteomyelitis will need veterinary attention.

EXOSTOSIS

An exostosis or outgrowth of bone tissue not uncommonly follows upon a periostitis. Long continued irritation to a part may cause bony growths, and concussion in some form or other is a common cause of exostosis. Among the more common forms of exostoses are splints, spavin, ringbone and some sidebones.

The treatment of these various conditions is dealt with under the respective headings.

BOTS

THE "BOT", as found in the stomach of the horse and commonly seen in the dung, is an intermediate stage in the life cycle of the horse bot fly (*Gastrophilus spp.*). There are several species of these flies and their larvae are the parasitic "bots" of horses which inhabit the stomach for a time.

Horse bot flies are yellowish to dark-coloured, hairy, bee-like flies which are not seen throughout the whole year, having a well defined seasonal occurrence which varies according to climatic conditions and according to the species. In Australia the common bot fly worries horses from January to April. It deposits its eggs on the long hairs

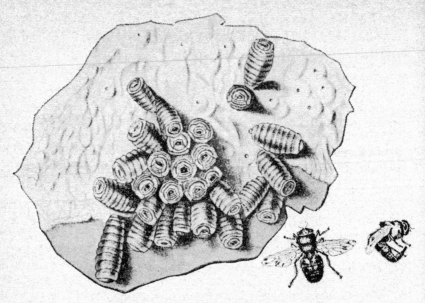

Fig. 3 Bot-fly larvae attached to the wall of a horse's stomach.
(From Diseases of the Horse, United States Department of Agriculture)

of the forelegs just below the knee and elsewhere on the legs, on the mane, chest and shoulders. Other species of bot flies deposit their eggs on the hairs of the jaw, throat and chest, while others leave their eggs on the long hairs of the lips and sometimes on the nostrils. The female fly hovers near the horse and darts in rapidly and deposits an egg which is cemented to a hair. This process is repeated. The adult female does not feed and lives from a few days to a fortnight solely for the purpose of laying eggs.

Horses resent the presence of the flies and kick or run away. This has given rise to the idea that the flies bite or sting, which, however, is not the case. The eggs of the common bot fly hatch in about seven to ten days and the emerging larvae cause some slight irritation which makes the horse lick or bite at the part and so the larvae reach the mouth. Here they make their way into the mucous membranes of the lips, tongue and cheek where they wander for several days. After leaving these tissues they may attach to the pharynx for a short time and eventually are swallowed and attach themselves to the stomach wall where they remain to maturity. The larvae of other species behave somewhat differently, but finally attach themselves to the stomach wall. Maturity of the larvae or bots is reached in eight to twelve months, when they detach themselves from the stomach wall

16

and are passed out with the dung, where they are commonly seen. Pupation occurs in the soil and the adult fly emerges in three to ten weeks depending on temperature.

Ill Effects of Bots

There is considerable controversy among horse owners as to the ill effects of the bots on horses. Actually their presence in the horse's stomach does not cause as much trouble as is commonly attributed to them. It is probable that they are harmful to young horses when present in the stomach in large numbers. Further, in horses of any age, the accumulation of bots in the pyloric region of the stomach near the duodenum can cause mechanical obstruction or irritation leading to closure of the pylorus. Occasionally bots may weaken the wall of the stomach where they are attached, leading to ulceration, abscess formation and toxaemia and, on still rarer occasions, bots have been known to penetrate the stomach wall and deaths have occurred from peritonitis. Heavy infection with bots may cause digestive upsets and unthriftiness.

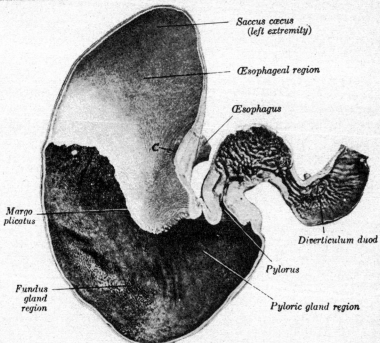

Fig. 4 Normal stomach of the Horse showing the different characters of the lining mucous membrane.

(From Sisson-Grossman, Anatomy of the Domestic Animal, 4th edition. Philadelphia, W. B. Saunders Co., 1953)

Bots do not eat away portion of the stomach wall, as is commonly thought by some horsemen who have conducted a post-mortem examination and examined the stomach. The left half of the stomach into which the gullet enters is lined with a white mucous membrane. Contrasting sharply with this—with no gradual transition—is the reddish-brown mucous membrane of the right half of the stomach. This contrast is so remarkable that a person without knowledge of the anatomy of the horse is naturally inclined to believe that one half of the mucous membrane is wanting as a result of some disease, or, when bots are found in the stomach, to assume that the membrane has been eaten away by the bots.

It is important to remember that unthriftiness in horses is more likely to be due to other much smaller internal parasites than bots, such as red worms, which cause a lot of trouble and are not seen in the droppings as are bots.

Treatment

An old and effective treatment for bots in the stomach of the horse is the administration of a gelatine capsule of carbon bisulphide in the correct dose according to body weight. As carbon bisulphide is very irritant and unpleasant, it must be given in a capsule as a "ball" or by stomach tube. The dose rate on the basis of 5 ml. (cc) per 100 lb. body weight is—foals 10 ml., yearlings 10 to 15 ml., adults 20 ml. The maximum dose for a large draught horse should not exceed 30 ml. The horse should be starved for 18 hours before treatment and for 4 hours afterwards but may be given access to water. Subsequently a light diet should be given for several feeds. Under no circumstances should a purgative drench, such as oil, be given following the administration of carbon bisulphide as this is dangerous. Other methods of treatment under veterinary supervision include the use of *Neguvon*, which has been found to be safe and effective.

Prevention

The protection of horses from the egg-laying activities of the female bot flies is difficult. The flies dislike shade and are not inclined to enter stables. With horses at grass, the provision of shelter trees or sheds into which horses may go during periods of fly activity is beneficial. It is not possible to protect the areas where the more common bot fly lays its eggs, but when the throat bot fly is prevalent, the under surface of the jaws and the jowl can be protected with sacking or cloth attached to a headstall. In this way the flies are prevented from laying eggs on these favourite sites and this may reduce the extent of bot infection. Washes of various insecticides are of little value in preventing the fly laying its eggs. Perhaps the soundest

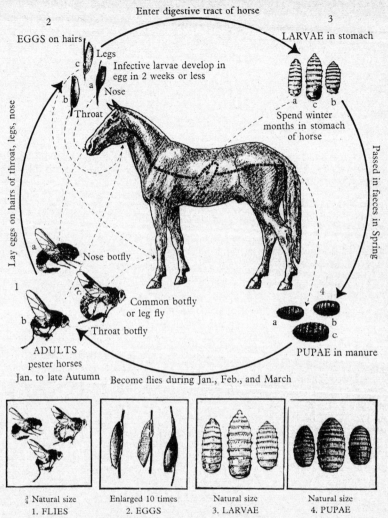

2
EGGS on hairs
Enter digestive tract of horse
3
LARVAE in stomach

Legs
Infective larvae develop in
egg in 2 weeks or less
a Nose
b
c
Throat

a c b
Spend winter
months in stomach
of horse

Lay eggs on hairs of throat, legs, nose

Passed in faeces in Spring

a
Nose botfly

1
b
c
Common botfly
or leg fly
Throat botfly

ADULTS
pester horses
Jan. to late Autumn

4
a
b
c
PUPAE in manure

Become flies during Jan., Feb., and March

¾ Natural size
1. FLIES

Enlarged 10 times
2. EGGS

Natural size
3. LARVAE

Natural size
4. PUPAE

Fig. 5 Life History of Bot-flies.
(*F. Thorpe and R. Graham, University of Illinois, College of Agriculture*)

measure is thorough grooming through the dangerous summer and autumn months to remove all visible eggs. Singeing is also quite sound, if well carried out. Frequent vigorous scrubbing of the areas where the eggs are deposited with hot water (100° F.) is also effective. This stimulates mass hatching and rapid death of the young larvae. No satisfactory repellent is known which will keep the female fly away from the horse.

19

BOTRYOMYCOSIS

CHRONIC abscesses and fibroid granulomatous swellings sometimes occur on the shoulder, the spermatic cord (scirrhous cord) after castration, the tail after docking and the udder, as a result of infection by the organism *Staphylococcus aureus*. The condition has also been seen in cases of poll evil and fistulous withers and may be found affecting the liver, lungs, spleen and kidneys.

When the disease affects the shoulders of working horses, it follows infection of bruised or chafed skin from a badly fitting collar. When it occurs on the end of the severed spermatic cord, it is due to wound contamination at or soon after castration, although the tumour may not attain a large size for quite some time.

Symptoms

The symptoms of external botryomycosis are the appearance of a small and, at first, soft swelling which slowly grows in size. The skin over the swelling becomes tense and the swelling may point, burst and discharge pus. The wound heals but the process is repeated. The swelling, while continuing to grow, becomes hardened and fibrotic, and granulomatous tissue is formed. The purulent exudate contains small granules similar to those found in cases of actinomycosis. Diagnosis is confirmed from pus submitted to a laboratory.

Treatment

Surgery is necessary in the treatment of a botryomycotic tumour, which involves removal of the diseased mass. Antibiotic injections are also given. Early operation is desirable.

BOTULISM (Forage Poisoning)

BOTULISM is a type of food poisoning caused by the ingestion of a powerful toxin produced by an organism known as *Clostridium botulinum*. It differs from other bacterial diseases in that it is an intoxication and not an infection, and therefore is neither infectious nor contagious. For the disease to occur the toxin must be present in the feed before it is eaten. The botulism organism exists as a spore in the surface layers of the soil from which it gains access to hay, silage, dry tussocky grass, vegetables and stagnant shallow water containing decomposing organic matter. In such situations, and subject to certain suitable conditions, the organism multiplies and elaborates its toxin. The conditions necessary are moisture, warmth and the absence or restriction of air. Moisture and warmth also favour the development of mould and, whereas ordinarily *Cl. botulinum* can grow only in the absence of air, it can grow in fodder exposed to air if it has a mould growing over it. Thus mouldy fodders are liable to contain the botulism organism. In a hay stack or chaff silo the fouling caused by mice or mice carcases is not infrequently responsible for the toxin in only a portion of the stack or silo. Grain may be similarly contaminated. In the case of silage, botulism spores may be blown into the silo and remain dormant until conditions such as mould formation favour their development. This is one reason why mouldy fodder should not be fed to horses or other stock. The organism may grow in dry tussocky grass clumps and commonly develops in carrion, including rabbits, birds and rodents. If this occurs near or in shallow stagnant water, it may be "poisoned" by the toxin and if animals drink this water it may be responsible for the disease. Toxic fodders are usually palatable and will be eaten by animals to which they are offered. Likewise, stock may graze closely on new shoots of grass over dead tussocky clumps in which the toxin has developed.

There are five principal types of *Cl. botulinum* known as types A, B, C, D and E, and, although the symptoms produced by all types are similar, the fact that differences exist in the toxin produced is important in relation to prophylactic vaccination. A vaccine prepared from one type will not protect against another type.

Briefly then the condition of botulism is produced by the presence in and the absorption from the intestines of a toxin produced by the organism *Cl. botulinum*.

Symptoms

The symptoms of botulism in horses, as in other animals, are those associated with the action of the virulent toxin on the nervous system. At first there is lassitude, drooling of saliva, a peculiar slow and very persistent movement of the jaws, and unsteady gait. Inability to swallow food is soon manifest. Eating becomes progressively difficult and drinking is only carried out with great difficulty. Often partially chewed food will be dropped or becomes lodged at the base of the tongue. As the disease progresses, the tongue hangs from the mouth and there is a mucous discharge from the nostrils. The horse stands in one place and there is slight swaying of the body and sometimes twitching of the muscles. Abdominal type respiration occurs due to paralysis of the chest muscles. The animal loses co-ordination of the limbs and finally goes down. There are no manifestations of pain but the horse struggles ineffectually to regain its feet, these efforts ultimately passing to a paddling action with both fore and hind limbs. The temperature is usually below normal except when the animal has become distressed from struggling, and is never high. Death usually occurs in from one to four days after the commencement of the illness. Some chronic cases last longer but very seldom does recovery occur. No characteristic changes are seen on post-mortem examination. The slight abnormalities which may be observed, such as congestion of the lungs and even congestion of the mucous membranes of the intestinal tract and abnormal conditions of the heart, are not due to the effect of the toxin. It is not uncommon to find food plugged at the base of the tongue.

Treatment

Little can be done in the treatment of horses affected with botulism. Skilled veterinary attention in the early stages of cases which develop slowly may effect a cure. Quick acting purgatives are given in an attempt to remove the toxin from the alimentary tract, and central nervous stimulants are given. Stomach tube feeding and good nursing are also recommended in mild cases of the disease.

Prevention

It is possible to immunize stock against the disease with a type-specific toxoid, which is a vaccine prepared from the particular type of organism present in the fodder. This is, of course, difficult to determine. Mixed type immunizing toxoids are available but are seldom used due to the infrequency of the disease. Generally, the main method of prevention of this disease is by careful feeding of horses and the discarding of all damaged or mouldy fodder, whether hay, chaff, grain or silage.

BOWELS—IMPACTION

See *Colic*

BOWELS—INFLAMMATION (Enteritis)

INFLAMMATION of the intestines (enteritis) is a fairly common disease condition.

Causes

In horses it is often associated with errors in diet leading to irritation of the mucous membranes of the bowels and infection by organisms which are common in the intestinal tract. Other causes are unrelieved impaction of the bowels or obstruction by calculi; eating of sand; twist in the bowel; indiscriminate dosing with irritant drugs such as oil of turpentine, or the ingestion of irritant poisons, sometimes of plant origin. Enteritis may also be set up by over fatigue, heavy hurried feeding, very cold drinking water, chills, sudden changes of food and internal parasites. Foals are commonly affected, when the disease is mainly of dietetic origin. Enteritis is frequently accompanied by gastritis (inflammation of the stomach) and may occur secondarily to some infectious diseases.

Symptoms

The symptoms vary considerably, depending on the extent of the inflammation and also on the age of the animal. Foals, for example, are very dull, disinclined to suck, exhibit a foetid diarrhoea which may contain mucus, have colicky pains and raised temperature and worsen very quickly. Older horses paw the ground, look round anxiously, crouch, may roll but lie down carefully, show continuous pain, dilated and inflamed nostrils, dilated eyes and inflamed eyelids, quick breathing, quickened pulse, high temperature, cold sweats, very cold limbs and ears, tender abdomen and a degree of diarrhoea which may be blood-stained and contain shreds of bowel lining. Increased thirst is also a symptom.

Treatment

Inflammation of the bowels is frequently fatal in the horse and requires skilled professional attention as soon as the condition is suspected. In the meantime, the horse should be placed in a well ventilated stable or shed and kept warm. A rug may be necessary and stable bandages applied to the legs are useful. The horse should be starved pending the arrival of the veterinarian, but a quart of warm, strained, well-boiled oatmeal gruel mixed with a quart of cold water may be offered frequently. Should professional assistance be delayed, 1 to $1\frac{1}{2}$ pints of liquid paraffin may be given as a drench, and blankets wrung out of hot water applied to the abdomen and frequently changed. Chlorodyne in $\frac{1}{2}$ oz. doses in a pint of water may be given and repeated every 4 to 6 hours if necessary.

In the case of young foals, attention should first be paid to the possible cause, which is commonly associated with an over-abundant milk supply from the mother. Frequent milking of a heavy producing mare, or reducing her feed supply, may be sufficient to check the trouble in the foal, if it is not too severe. In case the foal is eating the mare's dung, prompt removal of dung from the stall, or even muzzling of the foal, can be useful. Complete withholding of milk for 24 hours, and substitution of boiled water containing 2 oz. of glucose per pint every four hours, is often sufficient to effect a cure. Severe forms of the disease will require professional attention, which include specific antibiotic therapy and possibly also blood or other transfusions.

BRAIN—INFLAMMATION AND DISEASES OF

THE BRAIN may be affected by infectious diseases which directly attack and inflame the substance of the brain itself, or the covering membranes. This may be from bacterial or viral disease, but fortunately few of these horse diseases are likely to be experienced in Australia. Infectious diseases primarily affecting other parts of the body may spread to the brain and cause inflammation or abscesses. In some cases, toxins from infectious processes in other parts of the body may cause brain damage. Toxic materials found in some plants also have specific effects on the brain.

Depending on the area of the brain affected, and the extent of the damage, symptoms may vary from coma, drowsiness or paralysis, to loss of coordination, twitching or violent spasms and convulsions.

Other conditions may be caused by tumours, injuries, heat exhaustion or congenital abnormalities.

It will be appreciated that inflammation and diseases of the brain and central nervous system are exceedingly difficult conditions to diagnose and to treat and must be left to a veterinarian.

Certain of these diseases are discussed briefly in their appropriate alphabetical order.

BRAN MASH—PREPARATION OF

BECAUSE a properly prepared bran mash will be eaten readily by most sick horses and is therefore of importance in general nursing, details of preparation are now given.

Take a clean iron bucket and scald it; throw away the water. Then place 3 lb. of bran and 1 oz. of salt in the bucket, add 2½ pints of boiling water, stir well, cover with a folded bag and allow to stand for a quarter of an hour. Give when sufficiently cool.

BREEDING

See *Parturition, Pregnancy*

BROKEN-WIND (Pulmonary Emphysema— "Heaves")

THE TERM "broken-wind" is applied to a chronic respiratory disease of the horse due to a chronic alveolar emphysema of the lungs, and characterized by difficult breathing, in which the act of expiration is longer than that of inspiration.

In normal breathing the rise and fall of the flank is steady and gradual, but in broken-winded animals there is a double effort to expire the air from the chest. Pulmonary emphysema is described as an abnormal distension of the lung caused by rupture of alveolar (air-cell) walls in the lungs with or without escape of air into the interstitial tissue, which causes embarrassment of respiration. Failure of the elastic recoil of the lungs results in forced expiration.

Cause

The exact cause of this condition is not known and, whilst it is especially apt to follow chronic inflammatory conditions of the lungs, chiefly bronchitis, chronic coughing and excessive expiratory movement due to over-exertion, cases do occur in the apparent absence of these conditions. The condition seldom develops in pastured animals or in those fed good clean feed, but occurs commonly in horses fed dusty or mouldy hay over a prolonged period. The inhalation of dust from such hay aggravates any respiratory trouble that may be present and, in any case, brings about coughing.

Symptoms

The symptoms usually develop gradually. There is a fairly frequent dry wheezing cough which becomes more pronounced with exercise. A slight nasal discharge may accompany the cough. Following exercise, difficulty in breathing is seen, which is out of proportion to the amount of exercise undertaken. In the respiration characteristic of broken-wind, there is a double lift of the flank, and exhalation of air requires special muscular effort. In the early stages, the horse may appear normal at rest, but as the condition worsens, the typical broken-wind breathing is constant and is accompanied by a hollow cough. Still later a groove develops between the back edge of the rib-cage and the muscles of the flank, and the size of the chest increases so that the horse develops a barrel-shaped appearance.

Broken-wind is a definite unsoundness in the horse and reduces the animal's capacity for work even when moderately affected.

Treatment

There is no specific treatment for the condition, although certain arsenic and other tonics are said to be beneficial in early cases. In advanced cases, when the air cells in the lungs are broken down, nothing can be done to alleviate the affection. The symptoms in milder cases can be controlled by feeding only sound feed in smaller quantities at a time, dampening of dry feed to control dust, and pasture grazing.

25

BRONCHITIS

BRONCHITIS is inflammation of the lining membrane of the bronchial tubes.

Causes

The disease may follow a sore throat or a common cold, or be a complication of nasal catarrh, viral respiratory diseases, strangles and so on. It may also occur from the irritating effect of gases and smoke.

Symptoms

Dullness; loss of appetite; hot dry mouth; inflammation of lining membrane of nose; rapid pulse; quickened breathing; cough, hard at first, becoming soft and rattling as discharge escapes from the nose. The nasal discharge is whitish at first, but later becomes creamy and frothy and still later may be tinged with blood. By placing the ear to the side of the chest, unnatural sounds can be heard, such as wheezing or loud blowing sounds and crackling in the windpipe. The horse remains standing.

Treatment

Good nursing is of primary importance, and this includes a light diet, warmth, (usually by rugging,) and fresh air. Hand rub the legs until they are warm and then apply Newmarket bandages. Hold the animal's head over a bucket of hot water containing a teaspoon of Friar's balsam or eucalyptus so that the horse is compelled to inhale the medicated steam. Repeat every hour. An electuary is useful, especially when the throat is sore and one or two tablespoonfuls of the following may be placed on the tongue or between the horse's teeth twice a day—extract belladonna 1 oz., chlorate of potash 2 oz., boric acid 1 oz., glycerine 2 oz., honey to make 8 oz. Clean cool water should be before the animal always. An ounce or two of Epsom salts once a day in the drinking water, or ½ oz. of potassium nitrate (nitre) in a bran mash or in the drinking water for a few days is helpful. The horse should not be drenched as this will cause distress and may aggravate the condition. Modern treatment includes the use of sulphonamide and antibiotic drugs.

See also *Infectious Equine Bronchitis*

BRUSHING

THE TERMS "brushing" or "cutting" refer to an injury to or near the inside of the fetlock joint caused by the inside of the opposite foot striking these parts. The injury may be on the inside of the coronet.

Cause

The trouble is seen mainly in young horses which tire easily, or in old and out-of-condition horses. Some cases result from bad shoeing, especially the fitting of too wide a heel on the inside, or it may be due to the conformation of the legs, particularly if the toes are turned outwards from the fetlocks. The fetlock of a horse which turns his toe out is bent inwards as well as backwards when the weight is passing over the leg, and is thus brought nearer to the other leg, the foot of which may strike it in passing. The liability is greatest when the horse is fatigued.

Horses may "brush" with both fore and hind legs, but the trouble is more serious in the fore limbs as the horse is apt to stumble and may fall. Regardless of whether the "brushing" is slight, perhaps only to the extent of rubbing off the hair, or whether it is sufficiently severe for the skin to be cut by the edge of the shoe, the cause should be ascertained and an attempt made to prevent it.

Treatment and Prevention

The wound itself usually requires but slight attention, provided the cause is removed and the place protected from further injury. If infection is controlled, such a wound only becomes serious when from constant repetition of the blow, the part thickens. If this happens on the inside of the fetlock, it may result in an enlarged joint.

Protective boots and pads may be purchased, or a pad may be made from a piece of folded rug or blanket tied or strapped around the leg above the fetlock, care being taken not to adjust it too tightly. When turned-out toes are responsible for the brushing, special shoes should be fitted, of which many types have been recommended, the pattern depending largely on the type of work the horse is required to perform.

Special care should be taken with young horses shod for the first time and they should not be required to do fast work or be over-extended until they have become accustomed to their shoes and have obtained hard condition. Over-exertion of horses at any time should be avoided, especially if they are in poor condition.

BURNS

BURNS, with which may be included scalds, are not of common occurrence in the horse. Nevertheless they do occur and, when severe, can be very troublesome and may even cause death from shock.

27

Causes

The common causes of burns are exposure to actual flame, as may occur in a burning building or other fire; scalding from hot water; electrical burns, such as occur when a horse is struck by lightning or comes in contact with live electric wires; rope scalds; and corrosive chemicals which include acids and strong alkalis.

Symptoms and Lesions

According to the severity of the burn, it is commonly classified as first degree, in which there is a simple reddening of the skin; second degree, when there is skin destruction and the formation of vesicles or blisters, and so on. The usual lesion of a fairly severe burn in a horse is a diffuse oedema of the skin with or without small blisters and sloughs. In a very severe burn, the skin may be wholly devitalized and the injury may extend into the deeper structures and sloughing of the skin may follow

When a burn is caused by flame, it is quickly seen by the singeing of the hair, but when due to a scald by a hot liquid, there may be little to see for several hours or days. The seriousness of a burn often depends on its location. Burns on the shoulder and elbow or on other parts where there is much movement of the tissues, are difficult to treat.

In moderate to severe burns there is commonly absorption of poisonous break-down products from cells and tissues damaged by the heat, which may cause toxaemia. Further, burns in which there has been destruction of the skin are very susceptible to bacterial infection.

Treatment

When the burn or scald is at all extensive, the services of a veterinarian should be obtained as soon as possible, because the life of the horse may depend on prompt and effective treatment. When the pain is severe, tranquillizers may be necessary before local treatment can be attempted, and it will usually be necessary to treat the animal for shock. First aid home treatment of small burns which appear clean consists of applying a protective film of petroleum jelly or carron oil (lime water and linseed oil, equal parts). Tannic acid jelly in collapsible tubes can be used on minor burns, but must not be used for the treatment of large burns as it is toxic to living cells and may be absorbed and cause internal damage. Burns in which the skin has been destroyed, and in which there may be pieces of loose skin or other debris, should be cleansed by swabbing gently with mild soap and water, and then rinsed with normal saline solution (1 teaspoonful salt to 1 pint of boiled water). This is necessary to guard against infection. A mixture of triple dyes, available from any chemist, can now be dabbed all over the burnt area. The part should be kept covered, if possible with sterile gauze, and if the site permits, lightly bandaged. As a further protection against infection, sulphonamide dusting powder may be lightly applied to the burn. The powder should be used sparingly in conjunction with the other treatment.

The treatment of corrosive chemical burns requires neutralization of the chemical before the above routine treatment. A solution of sodium bicarbonate (baking soda), 1 dessertspoonful to a pint of warm water, may be applied to acid burns; weak acetic acid (equal parts of vinegar and water) to alkali burns; alcohol to phenol burns; and in chemical burns where the causative chemical is not known, the sodium bicarbonate solution can be used. Following the neutralizing washes, the minor chemical burns should be well swabbed with normal saline solution and a wet pack of same applied to the area and kept moist. Subsequently the wound may be treated as already outlined for minor burns.

Rope scalds can be treated with antibiotic ointments and further protected with a sterile dressing and a bandage.

Burns caused by lightning stroke and electric wires are likely to occur in irregular lines and, unless the horse is struck dead, the burns are generally not serious. If treatment is necessary, it is along the lines for ordinary burns.

It is important in the general treatment of burns to keep the horse warm, to encourage it to drink clean fresh water, to tempt it to eat by offering appetizing feeds, and to generally nurse it well.

CALCULI

A CALCULUS is a solid stone-like concretion composed usually of mineral substances and found in ducts, passages and hollow organs throughout the body.

Common calculi which occur in the horse are discussed under their appropriate headings.

See *Colic—Obstruction Colic* (intestinal), *Salivary Calculi* (cheek stone), *Urinary Calculi* (kidneys, ureters, bladder)

CANCER

CANCER is the term popularly used for any malignant tumour or neoplasm. These are unencapsulated growths characterized by the fact that they usually grow rapidly, destroying the normal tissue at site of the growth and infiltrating to adjacent lymph glands and deeper structures. They tend to spread to other parts of the body by the

29

lymph or bloodstreams setting up metastatic or secondary growths in new organs or tissues, including vital organs such as lungs, liver and stomach, with fatal results.

Carcinomas are neoplasms which are derived from epithelium (the cell covering of the skin and mucous membranes). One type is referred to as *epithelioma* and is not uncommonly found on the eyelids of the horse, particularly on the *membrana nictitans* (third eyelid), from where, if not removed early, it eventually involves the eye and spreads further.

Another type of neoplasm, known as *melanoma* because it is dark or black in appearance due to the presence of melanin, is seen in old grey horses (see page 126). The common commencing site is under the tail, above the anus or on the skin around the anus. Such neoplasms also occur on the head below the ears and on the neck and, more rarely, on the trunk. Metastasis occurs fairly rapidly to other parts of the body.

Cause

Many theories have been advanced as to the cause of the various types of neoplasms, which have been described as "the mad growth of cells at the expense of tissue on which they form". What causes the stimulus that produces a change from normal to uncontrolled cellular production is not known, and is the subject of intensive research work throughout the world.

Treatment

Well performed surgery carried out in the early stages of the growth before metastasis has occurred is the best treatment. Radiation therapy can also be carried out if there is no objection to expense, and good results have been obtained with certain types of neoplasms.

CANKER

THE TERM "Canker" is applied to a chronic moist softening of the horn of the horse's foot, starting at the frog and slowly extending to the sole and wall of the foot. This condition results from an inflammatory change in the horn-forming tissue which causes secretion of a serous fluid instead of the normally produced cells.

Cause

While the exact cause of canker is not understood, the predisposing causes which lead to the condition are generally known. Continued standing in dampness and filth, general neglect and injury to the foot, and faulty shoeing that removes frog pressure are some of the important predisposing causes of the disease.

Symptoms

The symptoms of canker are frequently not observed until considerable damage has been done and the disease is far advanced. The main signs of the condition are the offensive odour from the foot, the liquid secretion from the cleft and sides of the frog and the rotting away of the horn of the frog and sole. Eventually the frog and even part of the sole may be separated from the underlying sensitive tissue. Instead of normal horn being produced, there is often a fungoid mass. Deep in the tissues there is frequently a foetid cheesy material. As a result of the fungoid growth, the horny sole and frog and sometimes the entire foot become deformed.

Treatment

The cure of canker is no easy task, especially if the condition is well advanced. Surgery is indicated to remove the fungoid growths and decayed horn. A hot searing iron is sometimes used, but the knife is preferable. When the condition is extensive, this treatment should be carried out under a general anaesthetic by a veterinary surgeon. Antiseptic dressings are useless without first removing the diseased tissues. The surgery involves cutting away or stripping all the diseased horn and some of the healthy horn. The foot must be dressed regularly for some considerable time until it is certain that the new growth of horn is healthy. After the foot operation, the walls of the foot should be shortened and a broad plain shoe nailed on, which can later be used to hold dressings in place. The foot should now be held in a foot bath of two ounces of bluestone dissolved in a gallon of water for an hour. It should then be allowed to dry thoroughly, following which one of a number of astringent antiseptic dressings may be applied by dipping cotton wool or gauze into same and packing it over the affected area. A pad of oakum sufficiently thick to cause considerable pressure is placed over the dressing and held in place by pieces of tin fitted to slip under the edge of the shoe. The dressing should be changed daily, and the horse kept in a clean dry stall or yard and given light exercise daily on dry ground. The persistent application of simple remedies and great cleanliness are more important than any particular drug. Subsequently, care should be taken to see that the horse is properly shod to ensure ground pressure to the frog.

CAPPED ELBOW

CAPPED elbow is an inflammatory swelling of the tissues between the skin and the bone at the point of the elbow.

Cause

The injury is caused by a bruise at the point of the elbow usually by pressure when the horse is resting on hard ground, sharp stones, or in a stable where there is inadequate bedding. It may also be caused by the heel of the shoe.

Symptoms

Inflammation of the skin and rapid swelling, usually with a quantity of fluid beneath, are the early symptoms observed. This does not as a rule cause lameness, but the swelling may extend so that it not only covers the point of the elbow but extends to the armpit when there may be difficulty in moving the leg. The swelling usually subsides or becomes more circumscribed after a few days and may even eventually disappear. On the other hand, especially if the condition has occurred several times, a firm fibrous capsule may form and a pendulous sac may remain. In severe cases there is abscess formation.

Treatment

Early cases will respond to constant cold water applications, which may be given with a hose. These should be followed by the use of astringent lotions, mild absorbent liniments and gentle massage. If the swelling does not subside and continues to increase in size, aseptic aspiration of the fluid at the lowest point of the swelling is indicated. This should be left to a veterinarian who will also syringe out the cavity and may inject a corticosteroid preparation. In established cases an iodine ointment repeatedly rubbed into the swelling has been found useful in reducing its size.

In order to prevent recurrence of the condition, extra bedding should be provided in the stall. In the case of a horse kept in the open, a small sausage-shaped pillow about four inches in diameter may be attached around the pastern to prevent the elbow touching the ground when the horse is lying down.

Old chronic enlargements become very hard but although they are unsightly, do not necessarily interfere with the utility of the horse. They can be removed surgically.

CAPPED HOCK

THE CONDITION of capped hock is similar to that of capped elbow. It consists of a swelling over the point of the hock. Two forms of capped hock are recognized, the common one being due to distension of a subcutaneous or false bursa covering the point of the bone. The second form is due to swelling of the tendon sheath and serous bursa, more deeply seated in the hock.

Causes

As in the case of capped elbow, the injury is caused by a bruise at the point of the hock produced by blows, kicks or striking against hard objects. In stabled horses the damage is usually self-inflicted. Capped hocks are not common in unstabled horses. The condition often occurs when horses strike themselves during transit in railway trucks.

Symptoms

Swelling over the hock is readily recognized, especially if the hock is seen from the side. In the more common form, usually designated as "true capped hock", the swelling lies just under the skin, is soft and freely moveable. When there is distension of the tendon sheath, the swelling is firm and less mobile. Lameness seldom occurs in the common form of capped hock and, in spite of quite a large swelling, which is unsightly, the usefulness of the horse is generally not affected. When there is inflammation of the tendon sheath or of its bursa, there may be difficulty in movement and lameness is evident.

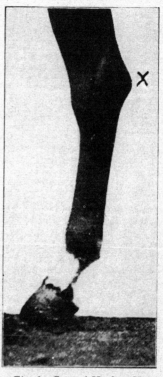

Fig. 6   Capped Hock at X.
(*United States Department of Agriculture*)

Treatment

This follows the same general lines as for capped elbow. Cold applications with a hose or ice packs, astringent lotions, absorbent liniments and gentle massage will reduce the swelling, but it is often impossible to effect complete reduction. Repeated applications of iodine preparations are also useful in advanced cases. Surgery is seldom undertaken because of the danger of interfering with the tendon and aspiration of the fluid is seldom successful, the contents being soon replaced. It is better to confine treatment to external applications. Pressure bandages and hock cap trusses are sometimes used.

CATARACT

CATARACT is an opacity or opaque condition of the crystalline lens of the eye or its capsule, which more or less obscures vision. Opacities of the lens are commonly observed in old horses and may gradually progress until the horse is blind. On the other hand, the cataract may only partly occlude the lens and have little effect on vision. White spots or opacities of various shapes occurring on the front of the eye, due to scars of wounds which have generally resulted from external violence, are commonly thought by horse-owners to be cataract. This is incorrect as cataract is confined to the lens. Cataract is not a growth but a biochemical change in the lens, and there are many causes. Although cataract occurs more commonly in old horses, it may be congenital and animals of any age may have small opacities. It also occurs in association with certain diseases such as diabetes.

Cataract is a serious defect in horses and is regarded as an unsoundness, although small cataracts may cause very little interference with vision. A veterinary surgeon is able to diagnose and determine the extent of a cataract with the electric ophthalmoscope, and this is important.

Whereas in man and the dog very effective surgery is carried out in the treatment of cataract, this is not usually practicable in the horse. There is no other effective form of treatment.

CATARRH (ACUTE NASAL) ("Colds")

CATARRH is an old term once widely used to describe inflammation of mucous membranes, particularly those of the air passages of the nose and throat and associated with a copious secretion of mucus. Today, inflammation of the mucous membranes of the nose is more correctly referred to as rhinitis. Acute rhinitis or coryza occurs in the common "cold", and is frequently accompanied by pharyngitis and laryngitis.

Cause

The cause is unknown but is probably a virus, usually complicated by bacterial infection. The disease is very contagious and, although horses of all ages are affected, it occurs more commonly in foals and yearlings. The disease is more prone to occur in the autumn and winter.

Symptoms

The mucous membranes of the nose are at first dry and congested. This is followed by a watery discharge from the nostrils and eyes.

These discharges later become thicker and of a yellowish-white colour. The animal has a slight fever, is dull, sneezes or snorts, but does not cough unless the throat is affected. The latter commonly occurs and may cause difficulty in swallowing. In uncomplicated cases, the trouble clears up in about a week. When there is a persistent cough and the animal has difficulty in eating and drinking, sometimes also discharging small amounts of food and water through the nostrils, pharyngitis is present. This may be followed by bronchitis, congestion of the lungs and other complications.

Treatment

The disease itself is not usually serious, but it should receive proper attention because it may lead to more serious disorders or become chronic. General attention to the comfort of the animal, isolation (because the disease is contagious), and good nursing are the main points to keep in mind. The horse's head should be steamed by holding it over a bucket of hot water containing a little Friars balsam, to promote free discharge of the mucus. Soft feed including bran mashes, if adequate green feed is not available, and fresh water should be provided. If the horse is not stabled in cold weather, it should be rugged. No attempt should be made to drench the animal. A few days of rest, fresh air and good feeding will be of greater benefit than most medication. If the animal is constipated, enemas of warm water into the rectum should be given several times a day. Sulphonamides and antibiotics are also used to check complications.

CHOKING

CHOKING is not as common in horses as it is in cattle, probably because horses chew their food better than cattle and do not usually feed on root crops. An apple is sometimes fed to a horse and a sudden fright may cause an improperly chewed piece of fruit to be swallowed. Choking sometimes occurs in horses that eat greedily and bolt their food, which becomes lodged in and fills up a portion of the gullet.

Symptoms

The symptoms vary according to the position of the material causing the choke. The obstruction may be in the upper part of the oesophagus (gullet), at the middle portion, or close to the stomach.

In high choke the head is poked out, there is great distress and the horse has an anxious expression. There is hurried breathing, frequent cough, excessive flow of saliva, sweating, stamping and the horse runs backwards. The lump can usually be seen or felt in the upper part of the neck. The abdomen rapidly distends with gas.

In middle choke the symptoms are not so severe. The chin is

drawn in to the chest, the horse hiccoughs and makes retching movements as though it wishes to vomit. The lump caused by the object can be seen and felt. The abdomen may be distended.

In thoracic choke the symptoms are less severe. Feed or water may be ejected through the nose or mouth after the animal has taken a few swallows. There are some symptoms of distress, fullness of the abdomen, cough, and sometimes retching movements. The obstruction will be encountered if a probang is passed down the oesophagus.

Treatment

Professional assistance should be obtained as soon as possible. In high choke it may be possible, if a mouth-gag is available, and with the aid of an assistant pressing the object forward from the outside, to pass the hand into the pharynx, grasp the obstruction and to gradually and steadily withdraw it. If this fails, external manipulation of the object upwards or downwards can be attempted.

Although obstructions may be pushed from the gullet into the paunch of cattle, such procedure is decidedly more dangerous for horses and should be left to a veterinarian. Whip handles or sticks should not be used and no attempt should be made to drench the animal, even with a small quantity of oil, with the idea of lubricating the object. Furthermore, do not allow the horse to drink, as it may cause the obstruction to swell, and if the stoppage is complete the water will only return through the nostrils. In the case of obstructions by soft feed, the saliva will eventually soften it and it will disappear.

Walk the horse about whilst awaiting the arrival of the veterinarian.

COLIC

THE TERM "Colic" is widely used to designate any form of severe abdominal pain in the horse. Through common usage, it usually refers to pain arising in the digestive organs. Whilst most cases of so-called colic do arise from derangements of the digestive system and are usually amenable to treatment, pain in the abdomen may arise from some specific disease, such as anthrax, and from diseases of the uterus, bladder and kidneys and also from calculi in the ureters and bile ducts.

Cause

It will be seen from the above that colic is a symptom rather than a disease. In this section, however, colic will be discussed as a disturbance of the digestive system.

Owing to its comparatively small stomach, and the bulk of intestines, especially the large intestines, the horse is particularly

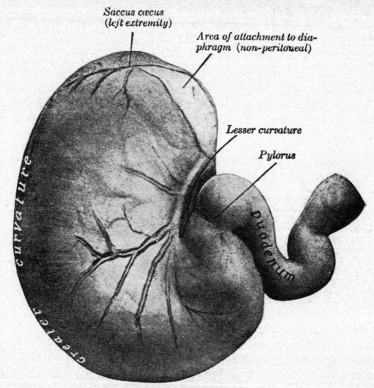

Fig. 7 Stomach of Horse.
(From Sisson-Grossman: Anatomy of the Domestic Animals, 4th edition.
Philadelphia, W. B. Saunders Co., 1953)

susceptible to digestive upsets. Most cases of digestive colic are caused by errors in feeding, faulty mastication or by factors which interfere with the process of digestion. To this, however, must be added the effects of overwork as a factor in the causation of colic. A sudden change in the manner of feeding; giving a large feed to an over-hungry horse; lush green feed producing rapid fermentation and gas formation; eating coarse indigestible material or mouldy, sour or fermented feed, are all prone to cause an attack of digestive colic in a horse.

Faulty mastication in young horses may be due to imperfect shedding of the temporary teeth. In older animals, the edges of the molar teeth often become so sharp that proper mastication is difficult. Indications of this may be shown by the horse dropping small balls of partly-chewed food out of the mouth, often referred to as "quidding". Horses so affected will often bolt their food without proper mastication, and this is likely to cause digestive upset through fermentation in the stomach. Removal of the sharp edges of the teeth with a tooth rasp will frequently result in the food being properly chewed. When a horse has developed a habit of bolting his food, a few big stones in the manger will prevent him getting too big a mouthful at a time.

Fatigue, exhaustion, and general weakness and debility will result in impaired digestion. Hard and exhausting work will have the same effect. Other factors which interfere with the process of digestion include heavy work on an overloaded stomach (especially in horses which do irregular work and are "soft"); severe worm infection; chilling due to exposure to cold when the animal is wet with sweat, and sometimes the drinking of a large quantity of very cold water.

The above remarks apply to the causes of colic in general. It is now proposed to describe briefly the main types of digestive colic, together with symptoms and treatment.

SPASMODIC COLIC

This is a common form of colic which obtains its name from the fact that there are intervals of ease between the spasms of pain. It is commonly known among some horse-owners as "water gripes", although it has nothing to do with the inability of the horse to pass urine. The pain is caused by sudden severe contractions of the muscular wall of the bowel. It might be termed a cramp colic. It may arise from chilling after heavy work or simply from overwork, from indigestible food, from a large drink of cold water or from exposure to severe cold and rain.

Symptoms

The pain begins suddenly and, although not continuous, is usually severe. During the attacks of pain, the horse paws the ground, stamps the hind feet, kicks at the belly, and crouches as if to lie down, looking around anxiously at the flank. The horse may straddle as though trying to pass urine. This last symptom gives rise to the common but erroneous deduction that the animal is suffering from an affection of the kidneys or the bladder. As the attack progresses, the pains get more frequent and last longer. The animal may throw itself down, roll and jump up again, paw the ground, kick at the belly, and become generally violent. "Rumbling of the bowel" may be heard by putting the ear to the flank of the horse.

Treatment

A veterinary surgeon has at his disposal a variety of drugs which will speedily deal with this condition. In the absence of professional assistance, quite good results are often obtained by comparatively

38

simple treatment. Walk the horse around slowly and, if possible, prevent it from rolling and injuring itself. In the interval between spasms, give by the mouth one ounce of chloral hydrate dissolved in a quart of water followed by a pint of raw linseed oil. Chloral hydrate, which is given as a sedative and antispasmodic, is irritating to the throat and stomach and must be well diluted in the above manner. The raw linseed oil will purge the horse. In addition, enemas of luke-warm water should be given every hour, using a piece of hose and a funnel held above the level of the back, if an enema syringe is not available. In cold weather, the animal should be rugged. If the above treatment has not given relief after a few hours, a further dose of chloral hydrate in a pint of gruel or a quart of water should be given. If chloral hydrate is not available, 2 tablespoons of powdered Jamaica ginger in a pint of warm water, given as a drench, will assist in reliev-ing the pain, but the raw linseed oil must also be given and the enemas should not be overlooked.

FLATULENT COLIC

This is a form of digestive disorder which is sometimes referred to as tympanitic colic, wind colic or bloat, and is associated with the formation of gas, mainly in the large bowel. It usually follows the eating of lush green pasture, clover or other legumes. Feeding a large quantity of green vegetables such as cabbages will cause the condition. It may arise from obstruction of the bowel. Feeding new oats or mouldy hay, or a heavy feed after a long day's work are other causes.

Symptoms

The pain is not as severe as in spasmodic colic, but is more con-tinuous. The horse is dull, paws the ground, makes frequent attempts to urinate and may or may not lie down. The abdomen enlarges, being most noticeable in the upper right flank. Breathing may be inter-fered with and the animal may attempt to lie down carefully but seems afraid to do so. Dung may be passed in small quantities and is usually accompanied by flatus (gas).

If the condition is not relieved, more serious symptoms may follow, due to a twist or rupture of the intestines, or the animal may suffocate from pressure of the distended bowels on the diaphragm, thus embarrassing the lungs.

Treatment

In the case of very severe distension, it may be necessary to puncture the bowel and a veterinary surgeon should therefore be called in. It is inadvisable for a layman to attempt to do this operation, which requires skill and care greater than that required to puncture the

39

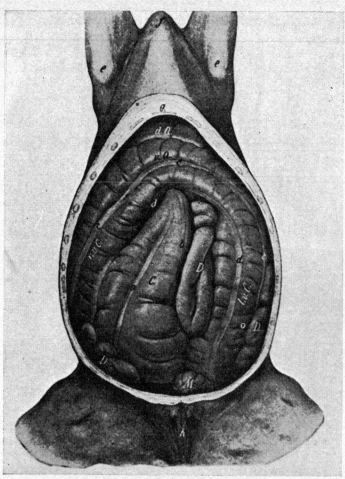

Fig. 8 Abdominal Viscera of Horse.
(After Ellenberger-Baum in Sisson-Grossman. Anatomy of the Domestic Animals, 4th edition. Philadelphia, W. B. Saunders Co., 1953)

paunch of cattle or sheep. A small trocar and canula is inserted in the right flank, and the canula is not left in.

If the pain is severe, one ounce of chloral hydrate in a pint of gruel or a quart of water should be given as recommended for spasmodic colic. The addition of a tablespoonful of formalin to the drench will help to arrest the fermentation. This should be followed by a purgative drench, such as a pint of raw linseed oil to which is added one ounce of oil of turpentine well shaken up, and shaken during drenching. If the condition has not been relieved in two hours, the dose of oil of turpentine may be repeated in a pint of gruel. The horse should be walked about and given warm enemas. Hot blankets may be applied.

A few days' rest and careful feeding on small feeds are advisable after recovery from a mild attack of flatulent colic.

OBSTRUCTION COLIC

This form of digestive disorder is usually more serious than those already described. It includes impaction of either the small or large intestine, and chronic constipation.

The common causes are overloading of the bowels, especially when food is hurriedly eaten; prolonged feeding on harsh dry feed; eating coarse indigestible feed such as wild melon vine, and so on. Other causes include intestinal calculi; displacement of the bowel, and tumour growths.

Symptoms

The symptoms of this disorder usually develop slowly. There is abdominal pain which may disappear for a day or two and reappear with more violence. The horse appears dull and the dung is passed in small quantities and is drier and harder than usual. The abdomen appears full, but is not distended, and the horse continually looks round at the flanks. Later the animal gets restless, lies down and assumes a characteristic attitude flat on its side with head and legs extended, occasionally raising its head to look at the flank. The

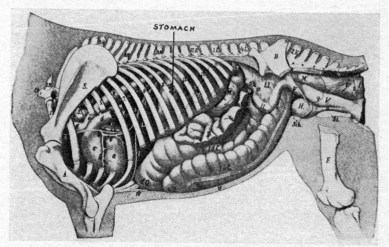

Fig. 9   Viscera of Mare—left deep view. To show position of stomach.
(*After Ellenberger-Baum in Sisson Grossman. Anatomy of the Domestic Animals, 4th edition. Philadelphia, W. B. Saunders Co., 1953*)

41

horse may remain on its side for five to fifteen minutes, then rise and may press its hindquarters against the stall or a fence and then go down again. On applying the ear to the horse's flank, no intestinal movement is heard. Pressure of the impacted bowel on the bladder may cause straining and frequent efforts to pass urine. When symptoms become more acute, the animal may break out into a sweat, the extremities are found to be cold, the mouth dry and the breath foul smelling.

Symptoms of obstruction colic may last for a week or longer and, provided auto-intoxication, enteritis (inflammation of the bowel) or rupture does not occur, the animal eventually recovers under suitable treatment.

Treatment

Efforts to produce movement of the bowels and prevent inflammation from developing, form the basis of treatment. The bowels must be stimulated and not paralysed by pain-killing drugs such as chlorodyne. Veterinary surgeons have many drugs to choose from to tone up the bowels and produce intestinal stimulus, and which when used in conjunction with other treatment bring about favourable results. Probably the best home treatment that can be recommended is to give the horse a quart of liquid paraffin, preferably by stomach tube and otherwise as a drench, to which stimulating drugs, such as ammonium carbonate 2 oz. and powdered nux vomica 1 oz., may be added and well shaken in the oil. This drench may be repeated in 3 or 4 hours.

Copious enemas per rectum should be given by a long nozzle syringe or preferably a length of hose. To be of value, these injections must be frequent, say at hourly intervals at first, and several gallons of lukewarm water should be used at a time. The nozzle of the syringe or the hose should be well lubricated with petroleum jelly or glycerine and passed up as far as possible without undue force. In my experience, prolonged enemas have given the best results when the impaction of the bowel has been due to balls of fibrous material such as wild melon vine.

Drinking water should be readily available to the horse, and the animal should be walked about and rugged if the weather is cold. Massaging and kneading of the abdominal wall may be of some benefit. It is necessary to persevere with treatment to obtain results, and professional assistance should be sought if possible.

Sand Obstruction

When there is reason to believe that the obstruction is due to sand, which may be indicated by sand in the scanty droppings, the horse

42

should be given up to a gallon of liquid paraffin for a large animal, preferably by stomach tube. Raw linseed oil should not be given. The paraffin should be repeated in a day or two, in smaller doses, say 1 to 2 pints daily for a few days. Then give 1 lb. of honey and a pint of milk warmed together, each day for several days. Otherwise the home treatment is the same as recommended for obstruction colic, long enemas being of particular value.

WHEAT ENGORGEMENT COLIC

Before farm mechanization, many cases of digestive upset occurred when working horses gained access to wheat grain. Cases still occur in light horses on farms. The digestive upset or colic which occurs is due to the production of lactic acid in the stomach, followed by impaction and acute dilation and inflammation of this organ.

Symptoms

In mild cases there may be only dullness, lack of appetite and sluggishness at work. In severe cases there is violent pain, the horse becomes restless, paws the ground, looks around at the flank and kicks at the abdomen. As the pain increases, the horse throws itself on the ground and rolls about. The respirations are hurried, the mucous membrane of the eye becomes yellowish in colour and the horse breaks out in a heavy sweat and may become violent. Temporary relief may be obtained by belching some gas or vomiting a little of the stomach contents, but, owing to its anatomical structure the horse cannot vomit freely and rupture of the stomach is more likely to occur.

Treatment

A veterinary surgeon would inject certain drugs subcutaneously to quieten the horse and then pass a stomach tube, wash out the stomach and then administer drugs through the tube. In the absence of a veterinarian, give as a drench by the mouth 4 to 8 oz. of sodium bicarbonate (baking soda) and 1 oz. of formalin in 2 pints of water. Follow this up with 8 oz. of Epsom salts and $\frac{1}{2}$ oz. of ground ginger in $1\frac{1}{2}$ pints of water. The baking soda (4 oz.) may be repeated in an hour or two if necessary. Allow the horse to drink as much water as possible. Enemas of large quantities of lukewarm water are of value. Chloral hydrate 1 oz. in a pint of thin gruel may be given as a sedative. Veterinary assistance should be obtained if possible, as the above drenches and other drugs are more easily administered by a stomach tube. Furthermore, a veterinary surgeon will give injections of antihistamine drugs to prevent laminitis (founder) which is a common sequel to this digestive derangement.

The common large roundworm (*Parascaris equorum*) is sometimes responsible for digestive upset and symptoms of colic. The worms may be so numerous that they become impacted in the small intestine, and the obstruction may be so severe that intussusception (telescoping of the bowel) and even rupture of the bowel may occur. Young horses up to two years of age suffer most from these worms.

Symptoms

The symptoms are similar to other forms of colic and may be accompanied by tympany (gas formation).

Treatment

If symptoms of constipation are shown, care is necessary in the treatment of the large roundworm when conventional methods, such as carbon bisulphide, are used. Under such circumstances it would be preferable to treat the horse as for obstruction colic and, when bowel movement has been obtained, to treat for the parasites.

See *Parasites—Internal*

VERMINOUS ANEURISM

The mesenteric artery of the abdomen is often affected by the accumulation of large numbers of an intermediate stage of a species of so-called redworm or bloodworm, *Strongylus vulgaris*. Whilst in the blood vessels these immature worms cause aneurisms (weakening and bulging of the walls) which interfere with the supply of blood to the intestines, resulting in digestive upsets and attacks of colic. A large aneurism may lead to rupture of the artery, resulting in sudden death of the animal.

Symptoms

Recurrent attacks of pain, resembling those seen in spasmodic colic, occur and indicate the possibility of verminous aneurisms.

Treatment

Very little can be done for the treatment of this form of colic other than to treat as for spasmodic colic.

The control of redworms by drugs found to be effective against these small parasites, such as thiabendazole, phenothiazine and piperazine compounds, is necessary to prevent the formation of verminous aneurisms.

See *Parasites—Internal*

CORNS

THE TERM "corn" is applied to a bruise of the sensitive sole of the hoof at a point between the bar and the wall. Usually corns occur in the fore feet, and more often in the inner rather than the outer heel. A bruise elsewhere on the foot is referred to as a bruised sole or frog. A corn is usually accompanied by haemorrhage and consequent discoloration from red to brown, a greenish colour, or yellow. There is pain in the swollen structures and the horse goes lame. In a moist corn there is a considerable amount of inflammatory exudate and discharge which may turn to pus. This is known as a *suppurating corn*. A dry corn is one unattended by excessive inflammatory changes which, however, may come later.

Causes

Corns are mainly attributable to faults in conformation, such as wide flat feet with low heels; long feet; weak feet with excessively thin horn; excessively flat soles and feet with high, contracted heels. Bad shoeing is also a common cause of corns which follow excessive paring of the sole, bars or frog. The type of shoe fitted may cause a corn. For example, calkins fitted too high destroy the counter pressure of the frog with the ground and cause undue pressure upon surrounding tissues, leading to the production of corns. Badly seated shoes have a similar effect. Direct injury from stones which may become wedged between the heel of the shoe and the seat of corn may lead to bruising.

Symptoms

The main symptoms are lameness of varying degrees, sometimes very slight but increasing with work, and at other times very severe. Tapping with a light hammer or firm pressure over the area causes great discomfort. In the case of a suppurating corn, the foot will be hot to the touch and the animal will flinch when that portion of the wall adjoining the corn is lightly struck. If not properly treated, pus may burrow through to the coronet to produce a quittor or suppurating sinus.

Treatment

The treatment of corns is not always satisfactory, especially in cases of very long standing. The normal procedure when a diagnosis of corn has been made is to remove the shoe, and then to lightly pare the seat of the corn to see if there is any suppuration. Excessive paring should not be undertaken, as this deprives the sensitive sole of its natural protection. Only in the case of a suppurating corn should the sole be excessively pared, and then only sufficiently to allow exit of pus. The important thing to keep in mind when treating an ordinary corn in a horse's foot, is to remove pressure. This may be conveniently done by applying a three-quarter shoe, which is an ordinary shoe with about an inch and a half of the side of the shoe, adjoining the corn, cut off. If there is a corn on both the inside and outside of the foot, a so-called bar shoe may be used. The use of these shoes allows a horse to walk without pain and prevents further injury.

Suppurating corns require special treatment. The main thing is to provide drainage. Warm poulticing or foot baths are useful to soften the surrounding parts, lessen the pressure and ease the pain. The latter treatment is also recommended for a moist corn. Useful dressings are a mixture of zinc sulphate 1 oz., lead acetate 1 oz., and water 1 pint (white lotion), or a five per cent solution of bluestone (1 oz. bluestone to 1 pint water). The white lotion mixture should be well shaken up before use. These dressings have both antiseptic and hardening properties. It may be necessary to syringe out a suppurating corn with a non-irritant antiseptic solution such as five per cent *Dettol* (2 tablespoons *Dettol* to 1 pint water) at least once a day. There are other equally effective antiseptic solutions. A leather sole may be applied under a three-quarter shoe, to protect a moist corn. In the case of a suppurating corn where daily syringing is necessary, several pieces of tin arranged from side to side and inserted under the edges of the shoe are useful, because they can be easily removed and readily hold cotton wool or tow, soaked in a dressing, in position. Systemic antibiotic treatment may be necessary in severe septic cases.

CRACKED HEELS

THE TERM "cracked heel" is applied to an inflammation of the skin in the hollow of the heel at the back of the pastern, and appears as painful transverse fissures having thickened edges.

Causes

The result of washing the horse and not thoroughly drying the heels, or any situation which results in the heels being continually kept wet. It was formerly a common condition in army horses picketed with heel straps on lines in the open.

Symptoms

The skin of the heel is reddened, fissured and tender. The cracks may become infected and suppuration occur, but more commonly they become covered at the edges by firm encrustations resulting from inflammatory exudations. As a result of this, the skin becomes increasingly thick and rigid. Lameness is present.

Treatment

Clip the area and wash the lesion thoroughly with warm water and good quality soap. Dry thoroughly. Dab on white lotion as recommended in treatment of corns and then apply zinc oxide ointment or zinc cream repeatedly.

CRIB-BITING AND WIND-SUCKING

CRIB-BITING and wind-sucking are acquired vices, both of which result in the swallowing of air by the animal. A crib-biter rests the chin on, or with his teeth grasps the edge of the manger or another object at convenient height, in order to get a firm purchase; he arches and sets the muscles of the neck, draws in air and gulps it down giving a characteristic "grunt" at the moment he swallows. The animal may even use a knee or other part of a limb as the point of support for the chin. A wind-sucker arches its neck, draws its head towards the chest, and swallows a gulp of air. It does not require any object to seize or support the chin.

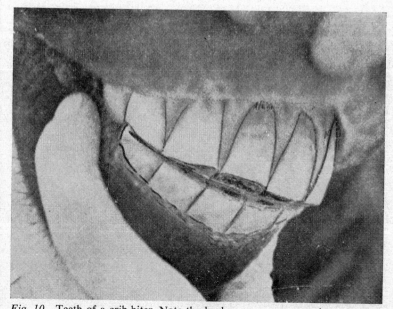

Fig. 10   Teeth of a crib-biter. Note the broken appearance on the outer part of the teeth.

(Bulletin 506 Horses, Ontario Department of Agriculture)

Causes

Varied are the reasons given as to why horses acquire these vices. It has been suggested that young horses acquire the habit of crib-biting from the irritation caused by teething. Idleness and boredom are also held to be predisposing causes. Horses are certainly prone to learn these two vices by imitation, and idle horses, particularly young horses, quickly acquire the habits if they are associated with confirmed crib-biters or wind-suckers.

Ill-effects

The ill-effects caused by these vices are loss of condition, indigestion and colic. Crib-biters wear down the front portions of the incisor teeth so that they do not meet properly when the mouth is shut and this interferes with grazing.

Treatment

Once the habits of crib-biting or wind-sucking are acquired they are never forgotten. There is no satisfactory treatment other than by the operation of myectomy (excision of a portion of muscle), quite an intricate operation which is claimed to be effective in a large percentage of cases. Many corrective measures are adopted to prevent horses indulging in these habits, which may be effective for a time, until the horse learns to outwit the preventive. For both crib-biters and wind-suckers, a broad strap fitting tightly around the top of the neck, with a small wooden or metal gullet plate stitched on so that it projects on each side and sticks into the throat when the head is bent, may be used to control the habits. There are various types of commercial cribbing straps, one of which has recessed metal prongs which press into the throat region when the neck is arched. Even a plain leather strap fastened around the throat sufficiently tight to make arching of the neck uncomfortable, but not tight enough to interfere with breathing, will sometimes be effective. A hollow tube bit, perforated with holes throughout its length may be fitted so that when it is adjusted suction cannot be exerted owing to the impossibility of completely closing the mouth. Another device is a piece of thick rubber tubing with a strap passing through it, fastened around the lower jaw just behind the tushes. It is not always effective. Care must be taken, when these devices are removed during work or feeding, that they are immediately replaced, otherwise the horse will take full opportunity to indulge in the vices. A crib-biter may be put into a loose-box with four blank walls and fed from a removable trough, which is taken away as soon as the feed is finished. This can be effective until the horse learns to use its knee or other part of a limb to rest its chin on, or learns the vice of wind-sucking. Muzzles of various types have been tried in the past in an effort to prevent the teeth grasping or leaning against the manger or other object, but they were not sufficiently successful to warrant their adoption.

Irrespective of what preventive measure is adopted, there is every possibility that the vice will recur as soon as such measures are discontinued.

CURB

THE CONDITION known as "curb" is the sprain of a ligament at the back of the hock, shown by a swelling which is soft in the early stage, about a hand's-breadth below the point of the hock towards the inner side. It may be best observed by standing at the side of the animal. Another condition referred to as "false curb" occurs in approximately the same area and is due to an enlargement of the head of the small metatarsal or splint bone, which may be congenital or be caused by a bony deposit. It can be differentiated from true curb by being bone-hard and situated towards the outer side of the leg.

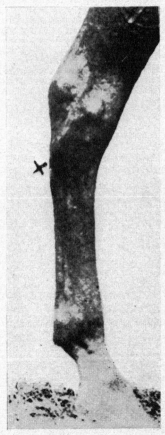

Cause

Although curb may be caused when any undue strain is placed upon the hocks, such as by slipping forward with the hind legs, jumping and so on, hocks of a certain conformation seem to be more prone to curb than others. Faulty conformation, as when the hocks are too bent ("sickle hocks"), or too narrow from front to back across the lower portion, appears to predispose horses to curb. A good hock should be large, and from its point the tendons of the hind limb should drop straight to the fetlock.

Fig. 11   Curb at X.
(United States Department of Agriculture)

Symptoms

Lameness usually accompanies the formation of a curb, when the swelling is more or less diffuse with varying degrees of heat and soreness. The horse stands with the leg at rest and the heel elevated. Later, the swelling becomes better defined, the prominent curved line is readily detected and the thickness of the infiltrated tissue is easily felt with the fingers. The lameness may then become intermittent or disappear completely, but the enlargement remains. A hock thus affected is less able to endure severe work and is more likely to give way with effort; nevertheless many horses with pronounced curb work well and no further trouble is experienced. There is a tendency in young horses for the curb to disappear, but in older horses it remains as a permanent blemish and thus reduces the value of the animal.

Treatment

In the acute stage rest is essential and repeated cold applications should be applied to the curb in the form of ice packs or water from a hose. When the inflammation has been reduced and the swelling has assumed better defined boundaries, blistering and point-firing are carried out and a further period of rest extending over three or four months is necessary. Veterinary surgeons have certain injectible drugs which are helpful. Special shoes, which have wedge-shaped heels, are beneficial in the early stages of curb.

DENTITION AND AGEING

THE AGE of a horse may be determined fairly accurately by the appearance of the incisor teeth. If any real doubt arises, an examination of the molar teeth is necessary. Nevertheless, even the best of judges may be deceived unless they have some knowledge of the conditions under which the horse was raised. For example, horses pastured on sandy soil will wear their teeth much more rapidly than those raised on loamy soil with better pasture, or those that are entirely stable-fed. Even the water horses drink affects the development and appearance of the teeth. When some doubt exists as to the normal wearing of the teeth, some idea of the age of the horse can be determined by its general appearance. In the case of an old horse, there are certain pronounced indications of age apart from the appearance of the teeth. For example, in an old horse the bones on each side of the nose "fall-in" on account of the descent of the back teeth as it gets older. With grey or roan horses, there is a whitening of the coat, and in the case of almost all horses some white hairs are shown, especially about the temples as the horse advances in years.

50

The depth of the hollows above the eyes is, to a certain extent, a guide to the age of the animal.

There are two complete sets of incisor teeth, temporary or milk teeth, and permanent teeth. The temporary incisor tooth is small and white, has a distinct neck and a short root which practically disappears as the tooth gets older from the pressure of the growing permanent tooth beneath, until its remnant is pushed out of the jaw. The permanent incisor tooth is, by contrast, broad, thick and yellowish or brownish in colour. It has no marked neck but has a long stout root or fang stoutly implanted in the alveolus (socket) in the bone.

THE PARTS OF A PERMANENT INCISOR TOOTH

The surface which bites on the food or on the opposing tooth is the table or wearing surface. Each permanent incisor has on its table a blackened depressed ring known as the infundibulum, surrounded by a distinct narrow light-coloured ring of enamel. This latter is easily seen and felt as it stands up a little above the rest of the surface. In the new tooth the infundibulum is very broad and deep, but with wear of the table it becomes shallower and smaller and gradually disappears. In some teeth, however, it persists for much longer periods than in others, the variation being due to the depth of the depression and the thickness of its enamel lining and also the manner in which the upper and lower teeth make contact with each other (uneven jaws). The blackening of the depressed area is due to discoloration from the food during mastication. As the teeth become worn away and continue to erupt, a central transverse darkish line appears on the tables in front of the disappearing infundibulum, due to exposure of the pulp cavity. The time of its appearance is variable depending on the method of feeding and quality of the tooth. The foregoing factors have to be taken into account when attention is paid to the so-called "marks" on the table surfaces of a horse's teeth as an indication of the animal's age. The shape of the teeth, angle of projection and several other factors are more important than the "marks" in determining the age of a horse.

The crown of the tooth is that part which is above the gum and the point where the gum and tooth meet is the *neck*. The *root or fang* is the part within the bone which carries it. It is hollow and its cavity contains the blood-vessels and nerves which nourish and sensitize the tooth (the pulp). Later the cavity becomes filled with a bone-like material known as dentine. All the permanent teeth in the horse are continually erupting, i.e., they are constantly being pushed out of the sockets by the slow proliferation of bone beneath their roots. (They do not actually grow longer.) This process is continuous throughout the life of the animal and compensates for the natural wear of the teeth. Thus, at first the crown, then the neck and finally the fang comes into wear. The "pushing-out" process continues in the absence of wear, and teeth which have none opposing them (as may occur when a horse loses a tooth in the upper or lower jaw) project beyond those in use.

NUMBER OF TEETH

There are six incisors, at first temporary and later replaced by permanent teeth, in each jaw. The two in the centre of the jaw are called "centrals", the next tooth on either side is referred to as a "lateral" and the outermost on each side of the jaw is the "corner" tooth. In the male, a tush or canine tooth appears behind the corner tooth on each side of each jaw when the horse is reaching maturity. This is a permanent tooth. Occasionally mares have rudimentary tushes.

There are six molar teeth on each side of each jaw, and they are numbered 1 to 6 in each jaw, top and bottom. The first, second and third are at first temporary and then permanent, but the fourth, fifth and sixth only appear as permanent teeth. Four other partially developed teeth, popularly called "wolf teeth" may be present, one in front of each first molar, but more commonly in the upper jaw only. They are vestigial teeth which were well developed in the early ancestors of the horse. They usually appear at the age of five or six months and generally fall out when the temporary molar behind is shed, and are not replaced. Occasionally they remain permanently in the jaw. Only the incisor teeth and the tushes will be referred to when discussing the age of the horse by the teeth.

FORMULA OF TEMPORARY TEETH

	Molars	Incisors	Molars	
Upper jaw	3	6	3	} = 24
Lower jaw	3	6	3	

FORMULA OF PERMANENT TEETH

	Molars	Tushes	Incisors	Tushes	Molars	
Upper jaw	6	1	6	1	6	} = 40
Lower jaw	6	1	6	1	6	

If the four wolf teeth are included in the permanent formula, the number of permanent teeth is increased to 44.

Tushes are usually absent in the mare.

52

Order of Appearance of Incisor Teeth

At birth the foal usually has two central temporary incisors in each jaw. Their appearance may be delayed for seven to ten days.

At about four to six weeks the lateral temporary teeth are cut and the outermost or corner teeth come through *at six to nine months*.

At one year all six temporary incisors in each jaw are in wear, the inner side of the corner teeth not yet grown up level with the front.

At two years the corner temporary incisors are well in wear, and all the teeth have well formed tables. Some care is necessary at this age in distinguishing between these well developed temporary teeth and permanent incisors.

At two years and three months there may be some evidence of the centrals giving way to the permanent teeth which erupt in pairs in both the lower and upper jaws. The gums may be red and swollen and the temporary teeth loose.

At two years and six months the central permanent incisors appear and at *three years* they are in wear.

At three years and six months the lateral permanent incisors are cut and at *four years* are in wear.

At four years and six months the corner permanent teeth come through and at *five years* are in wear, but not fully (a typical five-year-old mouth).

The horse has now twelve permanent incisor teeth (six lower and six upper) and is referred to as having a "full mouth". The tushes or canine teeth usually start to appear when the horse is four years old. When present, there are two in each jaw, with the ones in the lower jaw closer to the incisors than the ones in the upper jaw. At first the tushes have sharp points and edges but these gradually become rounded with age.

At six years the corner teeth are in full wear over their entire surface, and such wear has caused the infundibula (depressions in the teeth) to become more shallow, especially in the central teeth where they may have disappeared. Reference has already been made to the cause of this variation. The wearing surfaces of the teeth are broad ones, the centrals showing perhaps a tendency to become triangular.

At seven years the infundibulum has disappeared from the centrals and laterals but a trace of enamel may remain. There is a distinct notch on the upper corner incisor, where it overlaps the corresponding tooth on the bottom jaw. This is sometimes referred to as the "seven-year hook".

At eight years the infundibulum has disappeared from all incisors. Usually at this age, but sometimes earlier, a transverse darkish line appears on the wearing surface of the central teeth in front of the disappearing infundibulum. This is commonly referred to as the "dental star", and indicates that the teeth have worn down to the fang exposing the pulp cavity now filled with dentine. The shape of the table surfaces of the central teeth have become more triangular. The seven-year hook on the upper corner incisor has worn away somewhat or may have broken off. The "hook" completely disappears at eight-and-a-half to nine years and the surface of the tooth is again level.

At eleven years the hook reappears and the notch becomes successively deeper, so that by thirteen years it is very noticeable and usually persists throughout the life of the horse.

From nine years onwards it becomes much more difficult to tell the age with any degree of accuracy. The wearing surfaces of all incisors have become changed from the broad oval to triangular, the back of the tooth forming the apex of the triangle. As the horse becomes still older, the table surfaces become round. The teeth project increasingly forward and appear to be longer on account of the receding gums. With increasing age, the dental star, which has gradually appeared on the wearing surfaces of all the incisors, becomes a "spot" rather than a line and occupies the centre of the table surfaces. At ten years, sometimes a little earlier, a well-marked longitudinal groove known as "Galvayne's Groove" appears on the outer side of each upper corner incisor. It is first seen as a groove just protruding from under the gum and travels down the tooth as the horse ages. It reaches half way down the tooth at fifteen years, to the bottom at twenty years, is half grown out at twenty-five years and disappears at thirty years.

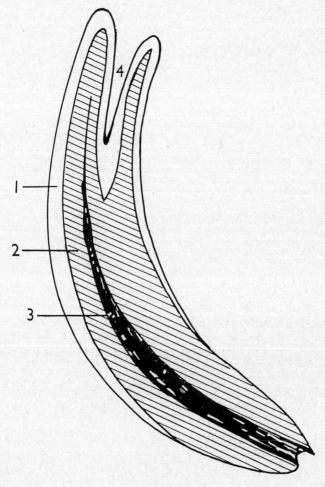

Fig. 12 Diagram to show the different parts of a lower incisor tooth and their relative positions.

1. Enamel
2. Dentine
3. Pulp Cavity
4. Infundibulum

(After "Animal Management" with permission of Her Majesty's Stationary Office, London)

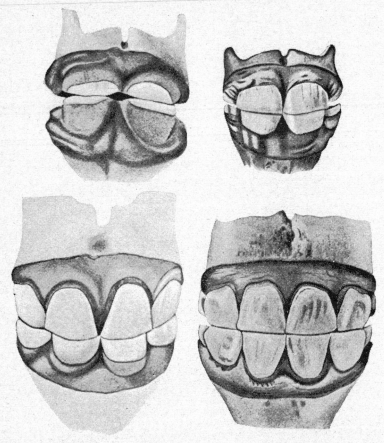

Fig. 13 (Above left) Mouth at about one week. The four central milk incisors are cut. The first, second and third temporary molars also appear about this time.

Fig. 14 (Above right) Mouth at four to six weeks. The four lateral milk incisors are through. The foal has now twenty milk teeth.

Fig. 15 (Below left) Mouth at five to six months. The front edges of the central and lateral teeth are worn level.

Fig. 16 (Below right) Mouth at one year. The corner milk incisors are well up and shell-like in appearance. The 4th permanent molars, four in number, are cut. The colt now has twenty-eight teeth, twenty-four milk and four permanent.

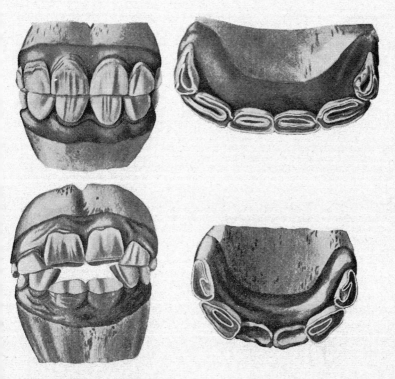

Fig. 17 (Above left) Two years.

Fig. 18 (Above right) Tables of lower incisors at two years. The tables of all the milk incisors are worn, the corner incisors have lost their shell-like appearance, and the fifth permanent molars are well up.

Fig. 19 (Below left) Rising three years.

Fig. 20 (Below right) Tables of lower incisors rising three years. The four central permanent incisors have replaced the corresponding milk teeth, and the first and second permanent molars have replaced their temporary fore-runners.

57

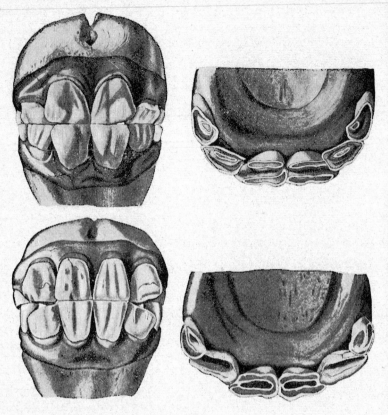

Fig. 21 (Above left)   Three years past.

Fig. 22 (Above right)   Tables of lower incisors three years past. The central permanent incisors are in wear, and the first and second permanent molars are well up.

Fig. 23 (Below left)   Rising four years.

Fig. 24 (Below right)   Tables of lower incisors rising four years. The four lateral permanent incisors have replaced the milk teeth, as have the third permanent molars, four in number. The colt has thirty-two teeth of which twenty-eight are permanent.

58

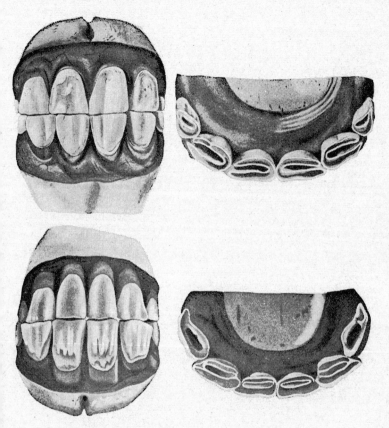

Fig. 25 (Above left) Four years.

Fig. 26 (Above right) Tables of lower incisors at four years. The four lateral permanent incisors are in wear, the sixth permanent molars are up, and sometimes the tushes are breaking through.

Fig. 27 (Below left) Rising five years.

Fig. 28 (Below right) Tables of lower incisors rising five years. The four milk corners have fallen out and are replaced by the permanent teeth. They are not on a level yet with the lateral incisors. The tables of the other teeth show more wear than at the preceding age.

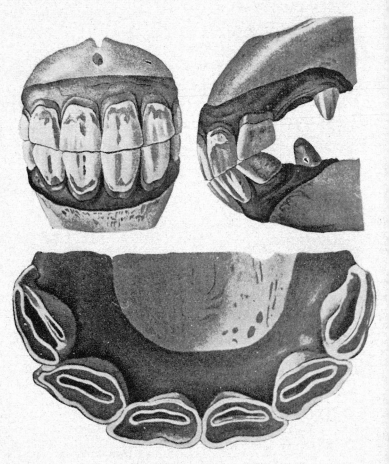

Fig. 29 (Above left and right)   Five years.

Fig. 30 (Below)   Tables of lower incisors at five years. At five years the mouth is entirely made. All the permanent teeth are on the same level in the respective jaws, although the inner edges of the corner incisors have not yet come into use. The tushes are now well developed.

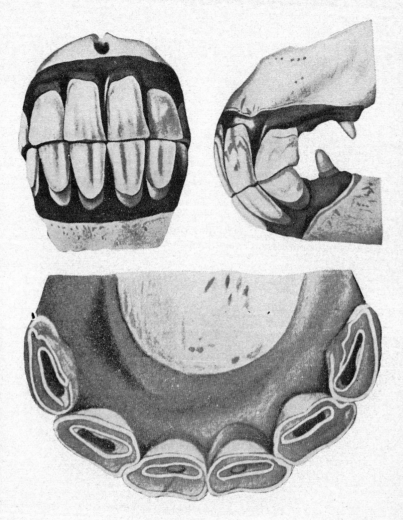

Fig. 31 (Above left and right)   Six years

Fig. 32 (Below)   Tables of lower incisors at six years. At six years the inner edge of the corner incisors is worn level with the outer edge. Wear has caused the infundibula of all incisor teeth to become more shallow, especially in the central incisors.

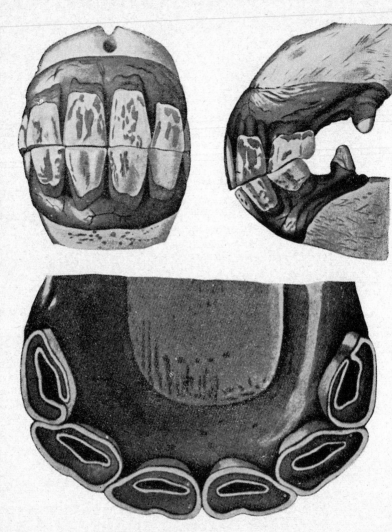

Fig. 33 (Above left and right) Seven years.

Fig. 34 (Below) Tables of lower incisors at seven years. The infundibula have disappeared from the centrals and laterals but a trace of enamel may remain. There is a distinct notch on the upper corner incisor.

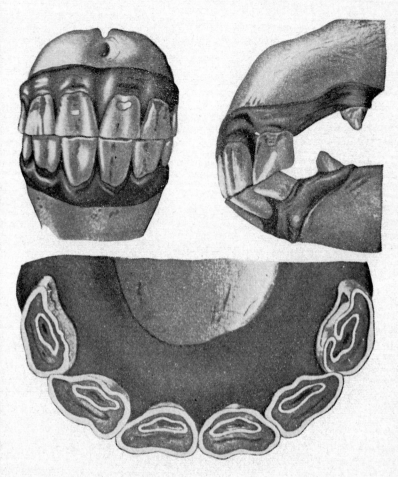

Fig. 35 (Above left and right) Eight years.

Fig. 36 (Below) Tables of lower incisors at eight years. The infundibula have disappeared from all incisors. A transverse darkish line ("dental star") is present on the wearing surface of the central incisors in front of the disappearing infundibula. The directive of the incisors is notably changed in both upper and lower jaws, and they are opposed obliquely.

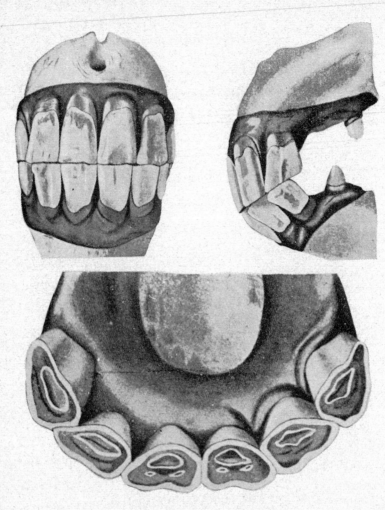

Fig. 37 (Above left and right)   Nine years.

Fig. 38 (Below)   Tables of lower incisors at nine years. The incisor teeth are more oblique and appear to be longer than at the previous age. A slight groove may have begun to show at the neck of the upper corner incisor. The dental star is more prominent. Upon the table the central incisors are round, the laterals becoming round and the corner teeth are still broad ovals.

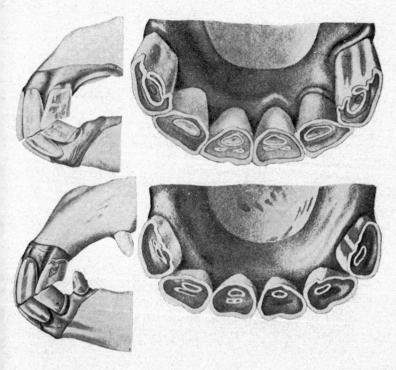

Fig. 39 (Above left)   Ten years.

Fig. 40 (Above right)   Tables of lower incisors at ten years. The incisor teeth have projected increasingly forward. The groove on the outer side of the upper corner incisors ("Galvayne's Groove") is more distinct, the tables of the laterals are round and the corners are tending to assume this form.

Fig. 41 (Below left)   Eleven years.

Fig. 42 (Below right)   Tables of lower incisors at eleven years.

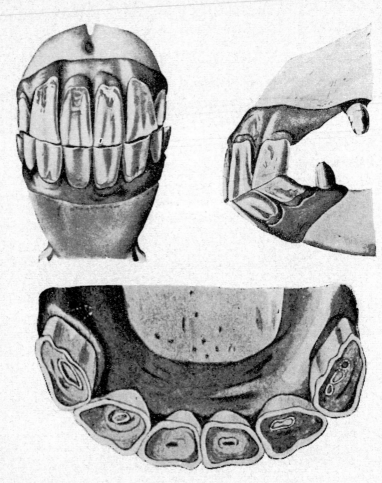

Fig. 43 (Above left and right) Twelve years.

Fig. 44 (Below) Tables of lower incisors at twelve years. In profile, the upper corner shows a greater obliquity than the intermediates. It carries a notch behind, and the interspace which separates it from the lateral incisor is more marked. The tables of all the lower incisors are now round, tending to be triangular.

The foregoing figures of the teeth at various ages are from Goubaux and Barrier as reproduced by the New South Wales Department of Agriculture in Farmer's Bulletin No. 87 "The Teeth of the Horse and its Age".

DERMATITIS

See *Nettle Rash, Mange, Leg Mange, Lice, Queensland Itch, Photo-sensitization*

DESTRUCTION OF A HORSE

WHEN it is necessary to destroy a horse, the most convenient and humane method is by shooting, provided it is done in the right place. It can be effectively carried out with a Greener's Humane Killer (if available) which is placed against the animal's forehead. In the absence of the humane killer, a pistol or small bore rifle may be used. Stand close with the pistol almost touching the forehead, and held at a right angle to the head. The head can be brought into convenient position by offering a handful of hay or grass. Aim at the centre of the forehead, about four or five inches above the level of the eyes, which is commonly in the centre of the "star". The animal will not fall forward but will collapse exactly where it stands, death being instantaneous, the bullet having passed through the brain. Care should be taken that nobody is standing within sight behind the horse.

DIARRHOEA

DIARRHOEA, usually referred to in animals as "scours", is a symptom rather than a disease and arises from irritation of the bowel.

Causes

Diarrhoea can be caused by sudden changes of feed; intestinal catarrh; irritation of the bowels from eating mouldy or musty food, irritant plants, chemicals and so on. Overwork, fatigue and exposure to cold wet conditions are predisposing factors. Diarrhoea may also exist as a symptom of a number of serious diseases, including worm infections. Persistent diarrhoea can be troublesome in the horse.

Symptoms

Frequent evacuation of loose stools, with or without pronounced abdominal pain, rumbling of the bowels, loss of appetite, weakness and staggering. Founder of the feet sometimes supervenes on persistent scouring.

Treatment

Care is necessary in carrying out treatment for diarrhoea and the cause should be ascertained if possible. The treatment of the condition, when associated with specific diseases, is dealt with under the disease headings.

When diarrhoea is due to faulty feeding, it may only be necessary to correct the feed. If it has resulted from some irritant to the intestines, a mild purgative, such as 1½ to 2 pints of liquid paraffin, should be given as a drench or by stomach tube. The diarrhoea is frequently checked after the purgative has operated, but should it persist, demulcents such as wheat flour gruel and milk, or lukewarm barley-water may be given. Chlorodyne, 4 to 6 drachms, can be given to relieve pain. Various useful proprietary preparations, such as *Kaomagma* with Peptin (Wyeth), are available from chemists.

Whenever a simple diarrhoea lasts more than one or two days, professional assistance should be obtained, because the withdrawal of large amounts of fluid from the body, as a result of scouring, may cause dehydration and it becomes necessary to replace this fluid. For this purpose normal saline is given by means of a stomach tube or injected into a vein or under the skin. Small tempting dry feeds, such as crushed oats and good quality chaff, should be given to keep up the animal's strength. Water should be allowed and the patient should be kept warm.

DIARRHOEA IN FOALS

DIARRHOEA is commonly shown by foals during the first heat period of the mare, which is 6 to 9 days after foaling. This is a simple diarrhoea which usually passes off without any treatment being necessary. On the other hand, foals not infrequently are affected by a condition similar to that known as "white scours" in calves, which is due to bacterial infection. Foals may also show symptoms of diarrhoea from other causes.

Causes

Foals are prone to eat dung and may also ingest genital discharges from the mare which have contaminated the udder and teats. The intestines of the very young foal are not ready to handle any solid material, so that eating dung and genital discharges causes irritation to the bowels and resultant diarrhoea. Another cause of simple diarrhoea, apart from changes in the mare's milk, is over-engorgement of milk by the foal which has been separated from its mother for a prolonged period, such as may occur if the mare has to be worked, or is taken away for breeding purposes. The condition may also be associated with an abundant milk supply resulting from the mare grazing on lush pasture or when given succulent feed. A predisposing cause is exposure to adverse weather conditions.

Diarrhoea caused by infection with various types of organisms is more commonly seen on horse studs where large numbers of mares foal, and infection occurs from contaminated foaling paddocks, loose boxes or yards. It seldom occurs when an isolated mare foals in a clean paddock. The condition is also seen as a symptom of other diseases of foals, such as joint-ill or navel-ill.

Symptoms

The symptoms of simple diarrhoea, unassociated with bacterial infection, are the appearance of offensive-smelling liquid stools and a reduced appetite. When caused by bacterial infection, the scour is usually yellow, offensive and may contain blood. The foal is dull, disinclined to suck its mother, the temperature is usually raised and the foal may show colicky pains. Some foals quickly become debilitated and dehydrated, have a characteristic smell, and die within a week. Pneumonia may be a complication and be responsible for death.

Treatment

Simple diarrhoea in foals requires little treatment other than keeping the foal warm and paying attention to preventable causes. If the foal is seen to be eating dung or bedding, a simple home treatment is to give 1 oz. of medicinal castor oil and 2 oz. of liquid paraffin. It may be necessary to muzzle the young animal.

If the milk supply of the mare is too abundant, she might be hand-milked and fed dry hay.

Kaomagma with Peptin (Wyeth), which is readily available from chemists, can be given to advantage.

Should the diarrhoea persist, or be associated with other symptoms suggesting that it is due to bacterial infection, antibiotic and general supportive treatment will be necessary to save the foal, but this should only be given under veterinary supervision. In severe cases, even a blood transfusion may be necessary.

DISLOCATIONS

DISLOCATION of the articulating surfaces of the bones entering into the formation of a joint is of rare occurrence in the horse owing to the firm manner in which most of the joints are bound together by strong ligaments. Generally speaking, a fracture of the bone is much more likely to occur than a dislocation, and this may occur in the immediate vicinity of a joint. It is necessary, therefore, to be able to differentiate between a dislocation and a fracture.

Symptoms of a dislocation

There is an alteration in the shape of the joint and in the normal relationship of the articulating surfaces of the bones. The joint is temporarily useless, and if a limb joint is dislocated, the limb is generally held off the ground and an alteration in the length of the leg is noted, it being either shorter or longer. There is a marked difference in the outline of the leg when compared with a normal leg. There is an alteration in the manner in which the joint may usually be moved; it is more or less immobile.

Dislocations are not always complete, that is, the articulating surfaces may be displaced but not separated, and the symptoms described above will vary. A dislocation may not cause much pain, depending on whether the displaced parts press on a nerve. Swelling and haemorrhage beneath the skin from damaged blood vessels may occur.

Points of differentiation between a dislocation and a fracture are the immobility of the dislocated joint as compared with the freedom of movement in a fracture, and the absence of crepitus in a dislocation (the peculiar grating heard as well as felt on rubbing together the rough ends of fractured bones).

The chances of recovery are better for a dislocation than for a fracture, but the treatment may be so difficult to apply that complications of a very severe nature may arise.

Treatment

The difficulties in the reduction of a dislocation are due to the contraction of the muscles and a general anaesthetic is necessary so that the muscles become relaxed and the various manipulations can be carried out. A variety of manipulations and equipment is used by the veterinarian to get the bones into place again. Special retaining apparatus is commonly necessary and must be kept in place for some time until the ruptured retaining ligaments are sufficiently firm to hold the bones in place. Valuable horses may need hospitalization for a lengthy period.

DISPLACEMENT OF THE PATELLA
(Stifle Slip)

THE PATELLA corresponds to the kneecap in man. It is situated in front of the stifle joint formed by the two long bones of the hind leg, the femur and the tibia.

"Stifle slip" or "slipped stifle" are the popular names used to describe displacement of, or dislocation of the patella. Frequently an actual dislocation does not occur, and the spectacular symptoms commonly seen in light horses, polo ponies and sometimes in foals, which have suggested the term "stifle slip", are due to muscular cramps which keep the patella drawn up. When the muscle cramp subsides, the previously immovable limb functions properly, but the muscle spasm is likely to occur again quite quickly. Rest, massage and the use of a stimulating liniment are indicated for this condition. When dislocation does occur, the patella is displaced either upward or to the side.

Causes

Dislocation of the patella can occur in any horse irrespective of age, but is more commonly seen in young horses. There are many causes, including over-extension of the leg when galloping, slipping when endeavouring to rise, a fall on a slippery floor, lack of tone of the muscles arising from weakness and general debility, and some-times relaxation of tissues due to want of exercise and use. A straight leg and sloping croup are predisposing factors. Foals, on account of general weakness of their ligaments, and especially if they are in poor condition, are more prone to dislocation of the patella than older horses.

Symptoms

The symptoms vary according to the extent of the displacement. The patella may be partially dislocated, fixing the joint temporarily and then, on movement, the patella will slip back into place. When the displacement is more severe, the horse stands with the affected hind leg extended backwards. It resists attempts to move it backwards, and, if urged to move forwards, will comply with a jump, dragging the affected leg behind with the front of the foot on the ground. The leg cannot be bent or brought forward. In lateral displacement, an en-largement may be felt on the outer side of the stifle caused by the displaced patella.

Treatment

In early cases of displacement of the patella, reduction can some-times be effected by moving the horse forwards and backwards and turning it quickly from side to side. Alternatively, whilst an assistant moves the horse forward a few steps, the operator pushes firmly on the patella in an endeavour to get it into place. If these measures fail, a long rope may be looped around the neck to form a collar resting in front of the shoulder. The free end of the rope is now passed around the back of the pastern and then through the rope collar. Whilst one assistant takes charge of the head and pushes the horse backwards, another pulls the foot forward with the rope, and the operator pushes the displaced bone forwards and slightly downwards into its place. When replaced, the rope should be tied to the collar to restrict movement for 24 to 48 hours. Stimulating liniments or a blister may be applied to the area with advantage. If unsuccessful in the above efforts, no time should be lost in obtaining the services of a veterinarian, as it may be necessary to give the horse a general anaesthetic to bring about relaxation of the muscles. Operative procedure may be necessary in severe cases.

DRENCHING HORSES

THE ACT of drenching is the giving of liquid medicine to animals by the mouth. To drench a horse, back the animal into a corner or against a rail fence; raise the head with the left hand so that the lower jaw is horizontal, or inclined only slightly upward; stand to the off-side of the horse and introduce a smooth-necked beer bottle containing the medicine into the mouth just in front of the molar teeth, in the space which is bare of teeth. Direct the drenching bottle well back and administer the drench very slowly, giving about 2 to 4 oz. at a time; allow ample time for the horse to swallow the fluid. The tongue should not be pulled out, nor should the left hand be placed over the nostrils, and there should be no interference with the throat. Water should not be poured into the nose. The only permissible action with the left hand, apart from holding the lower jaw, is to tickle the roof of the mouth with the fingers. Never drench through the nose. The neck of the bottle can be protected with leather or a piece of hose pipe for extra safety. Special metal drenching bottles and drenching bits can be purchased.

A small quiet horse can be easily drenched in the above manner. If, however, the horse is large and inclined to be fractious, a loop may be made in the end of a rope and this placed in the mouth just behind the upper front teeth or the tushes of the upper jaw. The free end of the rope is now passed over a beam above the horse's head and, after the head has been pushed up with the hand to a little above the horizontal, the rope is held by an assistant. If the head is drawn up too high, the horse cannot swallow properly and some of the liquid may enter the windpipe and so pass to the lungs.

Drenching should never be hurried and horses suffering from laryngitis, bronchitis or, in fact, any respiratory affection should not be drenched. Any drugs which are likely to injure the mouth and throat, such as chloral hydrate, should be well diluted.

THE STOMACH TUBE

The stomach tube is a much more convenient way of giving a large quantity of liquid medicine to a horse than by drenching with a bottle, and is generally adopted by veterinarians. It has many advantages including less disturbance and struggling; obviates the risk of choking; allows the correct dose to be given without wastage from

72

spilling, and permits of the administration of unpleasant tasting drugs which the horse normally resents when they are placed in the mouth.

The stomach tube is passed by way of one nostril, back to the throat, thence down the gullet to the stomach. This operation requires considerable skill and experience and should, for preference, be left to a veterinarian, who, with a knowledge of anatomy, knows exactly what he is doing.

The single stomach tube consists of a tube of firm rubber, nine feet long, five-eighths of an inch in diameter with a calibre of $\frac{3}{8}$ of an inch. One end is rounded and solid, the lumen opening about three-quarters of an inch from it on one side. The tube is marked at about fifteen inches and again at about $5\frac{1}{2}$ feet from the rounded end, these being the approximate distances from the nostril to the pharynx and stomach respectively. These distances will vary according to the size of the horse.

With the aid of an assistant, the horse's head may be extended and held in a straight line or may be left in its natural position. After lubricating with soft paraffin, the tube is carefully passed along the floor of a nostril into the pharynx. At this point involuntary swallowing efforts occur, and the tube is then passed four or five inches into the gullet. The operator should determine whether the tube is in the gullet by palpation in the left jugular furrow before passing it further. Should the tube have been inserted into the windpipe, it will be found to pass very easily, and the respired air can be detected by placing the end of the tube close to the ear. If this happens, the tube is partly withdrawn and then manipulated into the gullet. The successful introduction of a stomach tube into the gullet requires the assistance of an act of swallowing by the horse. When the tube is passed correctly into the gullet, it is quite rapidly swallowed and it requires only a little assistance of the left hand to push it foot by foot with each act of swallowing. As the tube approaches the stomach, the gurgling of escaping gas and the sour odour of fermenting feed indicate that it has not passed into the air passage. The medicine is introduced into the free end of the tube by a funnel. Care is necessary in withdrawing the tube gently, but firmly.

ECZEMA

ECZEMA is a non-contagious skin disease characterized by redness of the skin, the formation of vesicles or pustules which are accompanied by varying degrees of itching, and terminate in a watery discharge, with the formation of crusts. Eczema affects the epidermis or superficial layer of the skin whereas dermatitis affects both the superficial and deeper layers. The differential diagnosis of the two conditions is difficult. Although the causes of eczema are not fully understood, the allergy theory, at least for certain forms of eczema, is now generally accepted. The substances producing the allergy may be external on the skin or may be internal due to something eaten, and may enter the circulation by absorption from the bowel. There appears to be an inherited predisposition to eczema, but in other animals it is apparently purely environmental and associated with bad hygiene, soiling and the accumulation of dirt on the skin (lack of grooming), and excessive sweating. Certain leather preservatives on harness or saddle may cause eczema in some animals. Horses that are heavily infected with worms may not shed their hair with the advent of warm weather and, as a result, may become affected with eczema. The condition may even arise from an auto-intoxication due to certain methods of feeding or from overfeeding (food rashes). Still another seasonal eczema occurs during the summer months and disappears in the winter. This appears to be associated with excessive sweating and lack of grooming. The condition "greasy heel", dealt with separately, commences as an eczema when the heels and fetlock areas are exposed to mud and filth. It subsequently develops into a chronic condition. Another form of eczema, the cause of which is not definitely known, affects more particularly the long haired parts of the body, namely the mane and tail, and is characterized by a dry scaly skin in these situations.

Treatment

Because it is difficult to detect the substances producing the allergy in cases of allergic eczema, and other causes are not always easy to find, the basis of treatment rests in change of feed and even, if possible, environment. Good grooming, improved hygiene and attention to the general health of the horse are important in the control of eczema.

Antihistamine drugs are now used by veterinarians in the treatment of acute eczema. Local treatment consists of the use of mild astringent antiseptic lotions to control itching and the use of antiseptic creams, e.g., zinc cream, which relieve the irritation and promote healing. Much washing is harmful and the use of strong antiseptic washes, such as carbolic sheep-dipping solutions, should be avoided.

EMPHYSEMA

EMPHYSEMA is a distension of the tissues with air or other gases. Subcutaneous emphysema, which is an accumulation of air or gas in the connective tissues beneath the skin, may follow wound infection.

The condition is first noticed near the wound, but may extend further over the body giving the animal a blown-out appearance as though the tissues had been inflated. When pressed with the fingers, crepitation or crackling is noted. By contrast with oedema, pressure made by the fingers promptly disappears when the hand is removed. No special treatment is indicated for subcutaneous emphysema which usually disappears spontaneously. Attention should, of course, be given to the wound, and it may be necessary to puncture the swelling with a sharp knife at the lowest point. Hot fomentations are of value, and if the emphysema is on a limb, the application of an elastic bandage will hasten the process of reduction.

Emphysema also occurs in a dead foetus when efforts have been made for some time to deliver the foal, thus increasing the difficulty of getting the inflated foetus away without embryotomy (cutting up the foetus in the uterus).

Chronic alveolar emphysema of the lungs has been dealt with under "Broken-Wind".

ENCEPHALOMYELITIS—VIRAL

EQUINE ENCEPHALOMYELITIS ("sleeping sickness") is a serious infectious disease which at the time this book goes to press has not occurred in Australia, but against which every precaution is being taken to prevent its introduction. It is a specific viral disease of the brain and spinal cord which has affected millions of horses in the Americas and elsewhere, and has caused great mortality. There are three distinct types of virus involved, namely the Eastern, Western, and Venezuelan strains, named for the geographical regions in which they were originally recognized.

In recent years (1969-71) a serious outbreak of the disease caused by the Venezuelan strain of virus occurred in Central America and Texas (U.S.), when American authorities mounted a large scale control campaign. Viral encephalomyelitis is spread by various biting insects, chiefly the mosquito, and, particularly in the case of the Eastern and Western strains of virus, is transmitted from infected mosquitoes to birds. The virus multiplies in the bird host and the birds then serve as sources of infection for other mosquitoes which feed on them. Infected mosquitoes transmit the virus to the horse or man when feeding on them. In the case of Venezuelan equine encephalomyelitis it appears that the virus multiplies mainly in the horse and that spread of the disease occurs mainly from horse to horse. Birds may also be infected. Viral encephalomyelitis is a seasonal disease, occurring mainly in mid and late summer when the insect population is highest.

Symptoms

In general the symptoms of infectious viral encephalomyelitis in the horse caused by the three strains mentioned are similar but the prognosis varies. The following are some of the symptoms. Sluggishness and drowsiness are early symptoms in the developing stage of the disease. The temperature varies from 103°F. to 105°F. and may remain for 24 to 48 hours then drops to near normal. Groups of muscles about the head, shoulders, or flank may be seen to twitch spasmodically. With the progress the disease the animal stands dejectedly and moves with an awkward staggering gait. Some animals may blunder blindly into obstructions in their path. In some cases there is extreme sensitiveness as shown by flinching at the slightest touch or by jerking muscular contractions when disturbed. The dejectedly sleepy horse may show a momentary interest in feed or water, only soon to lapse into a stupor with unchewed food in the mouth, or water trickling from the mouth or nostrils.

Treatment

This is difficult and is essentially a matter for a veterinarian.

Control

Very little can be done to control insect vectors such as mosquitoes, and because of this method of spread of the disease and the high incidence in wild birds, especially in relation to the Eastern and Western types, complete eradication of the disease once it has been introduced into an area appears to be impossible. Annual immunization of horses, using vaccines prepared from the appropriate strains of the virus, is the most satisfactory way of controlling the disease.

Because man is susceptible to the causative virus the possible introduction of the disease is also of considerable public health significance.

EQUINE INFECTIOUS ANAEMIA (Swamp Fever)

EQUINE infectious anaemia or swamp fever, as it is commonly called, is an acute or chronic contagious disease of the horse, ass and mule, characterized principally by intermittent fever, marked depression, loss of condition, oedema and anaemia. The disease is found in most countries, including Australia, where it was first diagnosed in 1959, but it would appear to have been present and fairly widely distributed before then. The disease occurs most commonly in low lying and swampy country, particularly during the summer months, although chronic cases persist throughout the year.

Cause

The disease is caused by a specific virus which persists in the body of an affected animal for many years and is eliminated in the milk,

76

semen, nasal and eye secretions, and in the urine and dung. Although essentially a disease of members of the horse family, possible experimental transmission to pigs and sheep has been recorded, and cases have been reported in humans with anaemia as the main symptom.

Methods of Transmission

Biting flies, mosquitoes and other blood sucking parasites mechanically transmit the virus from a "carrier" animal to healthy horses. This would appear to be the reason why the disease spreads more readily in spring and summer and in swampy areas. Contaminated food and water may be a source of spread of the disease, but relatively large amounts of virus must be ingested to cause infection. Stabling of a "carrier" animal with healthy horses, especially over a period, will spread the infection. Foals sucking infected mothers can contract the disease through the milk, and a stallion could transmit the disease to mares at service. Infection can also be spread by contaminated surgical or tattoo instruments or the use of unsterilized hypodermic needles, when horses are being inoculated against some other disease.

Symptoms

The incubation period of the disease in natural outbreaks is generally considered to be two to four weeks. The symptoms vary greatly depending largely on the form of the disease. Ordinarily the disease appears to spread slowly, occurring in isolated cases, but it may occur as an epidemic in a large group of susceptible horses following the introduction of "carriers", when circumstances are favourable for its transmission. The disease may occur either as an acute rapidly fatal disease with continuous or intermittent high fever, the temperature ranging to 106° F., with great prostration and death within a few days, or the attacks of fever may gradually decrease in intensity and frequency, and the disease becomes sub-acute or chronic. Usually the disease begins in the sub-acute form and the symptoms come on more gradually, being less severe intermittent fever attacks; depression; lack of appetite; progressive weakness; loss of condition; dropsical swellings of the lower portions of the body and legs; jaundice; pin-point haemorrhages on the mucous membranes of the eyes, nose and mouth, and later signs of anaemia. There may be a slight watery discharge from the eyes and nose and, if the weather is warm, profuse sweating occurs. Frequent urination may be noted and a foetid, watery diarrhoea is sometimes seen. It is common for animals to recover from this sub-acute form of the disease over a period of about three weeks and then to suffer a relapse. The symptoms shown, however, are usually less severe, although an animal may die during such a

77

relapse. Subsequent attacks become less frequent, the animal finally developing into a chronic case or a recovered "carrier".

During the attacks of fever and immediately afterwards, there is destruction of red blood corpuscles which causes the anaemia, as shown by paleness of the visible mucous membranes, e.g., the eyes and inside the nose. There is also considerable enlargement of the spleen, which at post-mortem examination is seen to be very dark in colour.

In general, the chronic form of the disease is manifested by unthriftiness, rough coat, loss of weight, sluggishness and general weakness. Symptoms of anaemia may be evident as shown by pallor of the visible mucous membranes. Horses affected with this form of the disease eat well, but in spite of this do not put on weight, and are subject to recurrent febrile attacks. Death may occur during one of these attacks, or the animal may subsequently die from exhaustion.

The disease may exist in a form in which no clinical symptoms are shown, yet the affected animal carries virulent virus in the blood-stream and is a constant source of infection to other horses through the insect vector.

The mortality rate from this disease is high and pregnant mares may abort.

Diagnosis

Definite diagnosis of the disease is difficult as it may be confused with a number of other diseases, especially in acute cases. The only reliable way is by transmission tests at a laboratory, thus calling for veterinary attention. The disease may be suspected when a number of horses in a horse establishment or on a property suddenly become sick for no apparent reason and develop symptoms as described.

Treatment

No specific treatment or vaccination procedure has been developed for the disease. Many chemicals, drugs and antibiotics have been tried, but with poor results and no lasting value.

Control

Equine infectious anaemia is a notifiable disease in all States of the Commonwealth of Australia, and suspected cases should be reported to the nearest official veterinary officer in order that suitable control measures can be carried out. Attempts should be made to control flies and mosquitoes and care taken that any surgical instruments, including tattooing outfits and hypodermic syringes and needles, are properly sterilized. The introduction of horses from known infected areas should be avoided.

78

EYE—FOREIGN BODIES IN

FOREIGN bodies, such as oat husks, chaff and other material of plant origin occasionally enter the horse's eye, and not uncommonly mud or grit enters the eyes during racing. Usually the foreign bodies become lodged on the internal surface of the eyelids or in the conjunctival sacs, but sometimes they penetrate more deeply. The irritation causes an acute conjunctivitis, the eye is half closed and it weeps. The third eyelid or haw may protrude across the eye and the animal avoids bright light. Complications occur if the foreign body is not speedily removed.

Treatment

Because the eye is so extremely sensitive and the animal resists examination, it is often a difficult task to remove a foreign body. It is, therefore, advisable to obtain professional assistance and have the foreign body removed under a local anaesthetic. If a veterinarian is not available, it may be possible, with the aid of a twitch, to syringe out the eye with normal saline solution (1 oz. of salt to a pint of boiled water) or with a lukewarm boracic acid solution. This may in itself dislodge the foreign body but, if not, and the object can be seen, it may often be removed with the corner of a clean handkerchief or the little finger covered with the handkerchief or a piece of fine linen. A feather dipped in castor oil or glycerine and used against the hackles can also be used. A fractious horse will necessarily have to be thrown. After the foreign body has been removed, the eye should be syringed out again with normal saline or some other appropriate eye-wash used, and such syringing continued for a day or so to control further infection. Antibiotic ophthalmic ointments which are readily available at chemists are convenient to use. It is very important that the foreign body be removed as soon as possible, otherwise ulceration of the cornea may occur and lead to loss of sight.

Occlusion of the lacrimal duct, through which the tears escape from the conjunctival sac into the nasal chambers, may also occur as a result of its obstruction by a foreign object such as a seed, and there are other causes. Such an obstruction will require veterinary attention.

EYE—CONJUNCTIVITIS

CONJUNCTIVITIS, or inflammation of the conjunctiva, is a common condition amongst animals and is probably the most common condition affecting the eye of the horse. As a rule, it is not in itself a serious disease, but it may give rise to serious complications such as ulceration of the cornea, which may be incurable and lead to loss of sight. Conjunctivitis, with accompanying eye discharges, occurs in association with a number of febrile infectious diseases such as strangles and influenza.

Cause

Apart from conjunctivitis associated with febrile infectious diseases, which usually clear up if the disease is overcome, inflammation of the conjunctiva occurs from blows or other injuries to the eye; from the presence of foreign bodies in the eye, such as sand, pollen, seeds, oat husks, chaff, lime and irritant gases. All these agents act as exciting causes, the direct cause of the inflammation being the activity of organisms which are already present on the moist surface of the conjunctiva or which are blown on to it from the air. Flies may also carry infection to the eyes.

Specific bacterial and viral infections of the eyes, and allergies, also cause conjunctivitis.

Symptoms

The first symptoms of conjunctivitis are redness and swelling of the lining membrane of the eyelids, a watery discharge and a tendency for the animal to keep the eyelids closed and to seek the shade. Later the watery discharge thickens and may become purulent, blister the surrounding skin and mat the hair together. The eye may be kept completely closed or only slightly opened, or the discharge may glue the eyelids together. An inflammation of the conjunctival membrane, or of the cornea beneath it, may result in an opacity of a part or the whole of the front of the eye. This may partially blind the animal for a time.

Treatment

It is important to allay inflammation and control infection quickly to avoid structural alterations to the eye. Discharges should be cleaned away with warm water to which a little boracic acid has been added and a search then made for any foreign body which may have become lodged in the eye. If found, action should be taken along the lines already indicated under "Foreign Bodies in the Eye". Frequent irrigation of the eye is desirable, using normal saline solution (1 teaspoonful of salt to a pint of boiled water), either by means of a small syringe, or a piece of cotton wool soaked in the solution and squeezed into the corner of the eye. Irritant eye lotions should not be used. A range of antibiotic preparations are, however, available as eye drops, creams and pellets which can be used to advantage, but preferably under veterinary supervision. The horse should have access to shade or be kept in a loose-box. A piece of cloth attached to a headstall and hung over the affected eye will shade it from light.

EYE—KERATITIS

KERATITIS means inflammation and ulceration of the cornea, the clear part of the front of the eye. It not infrequently supervenes on neglected cases of conjunctivitis, the basic causes being the same.

Symptoms

The early symptoms are similar to those of conjunctivitis, but as the pain is more intense than in the latter condition, the horse is inclined to keep the eye permanently closed and examination is carried out with some difficulty. A close inspection shows the surface of the cornea to be duller than usual, the dullness varying from a slight haze to a bluish appearance. Later the blood vessels around the margins of the eye are congested and begin to spread over the eye when the white of the eye appears blood-shot. This condition is usually associated with a discharge of pus from the eye. Still later, irregularities occur on the cornea and commonly a small projection may be seen on the surface of the cornea, usually greyish in colour

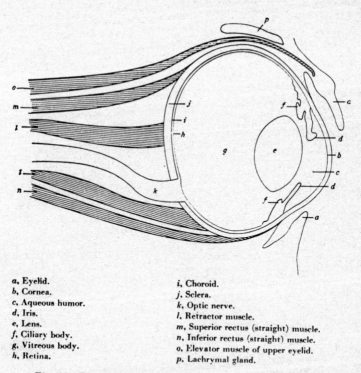

a, Eyelid.	*i*, Choroid.
b, Cornea.	*j*, Sclera.
c, Aqueous humor.	*k*, Optic nerve.
d, Iris.	*l*, Retractor muscle.
e, Lens.	*m*, Superior rectus (straight) muscle.
f, Ciliary body.	*n*, Inferior rectus (straight) muscle.
g, Vitreous body.	*o*, Elevator muscle of upper eyelid.
h, Retina.	*p*, Lachrymal gland.

Fig. 45 Diagrammatic vertical section through horse's eye.

(*Diseases of the Horse. United States Department of Agriculture*)

or tinged with pink. This indicates that ulceration has destroyed the wall of the cornea and the pressure of the contents of the eyeball has pressed outwards the membrane which lines it on the inside. Recovery may occur at this stage, and the eye revert to normal, although a slight film may remain. In severe cases, continued ulceration causes the membrane to rupture, the fluid content escapes through the hole in the cornea, and the front of the eyeball collapses, causing permanent loss of sight in the affected eye.

Keratitis is frequently accompanied by fever and constitutional disturbance, probably occasioned by pain and fear.

Treatment

Antiseptic treatment as recommended for conjunctivitis will often check the development of this condition if meticulously carried out. Once it has developed, treatment should be left to a veterinarian. Antibiotic and sulphonamide preparations are used and veterinary surgeons often use corticosteroids in conjunction with them. The risk of failure of home treatment is not worthwhile when the sight of the horse's eye is at stake.

EYE—HABRONEMIC CONJUNCTIVITIS

HOUSE flies, bush flies and stable flies act as intermediate hosts of certain species of stomach worms of horses of the genus *Habronema*. Infected flies feeding on the borders of the horse's eyelids, especially at the inner corner of the eye, may deposit *Habronema* larvae, which penetrate the mucous membrane. This causes considerable irritation, followed by a persistent conjunctivitis and frequently the development of a nodular ulcer. On the third eyelid the nodule may be as big as a quarter of an inch in diameter. A profuse watery and sometimes purulent discharge from the eye attracts more flies, thus aggravating the condition. These *Habronema* nodules are frequently mistaken for cancer of the eye (see *Tumours*) and indeed may develop into the malignant condition.

Treatment

Habronemic conjunctivitis does not respond to the usual treatments for conjunctivitis. Daily applications of pure glycerine are recommended. It may be necessary to remove the nodules surgically. Repellants applied around the eyes are not very satisfactory in keeping the flies away. Heavy fly veils should be fitted to headstalls on the horse, and attention paid to disposal of manure to destroy the worm eggs and so prevent hatching of the flies.

EYE—PERIODIC OPHTHALMIA

PERIODIC ophthalmia has been recognized as a disease of horses and mules since ancient times and, although much study has been carried out, the cause of the disease has not yet been definitely determined. The latest theory is that it is associated with infection by a particular organism of the genus *Leptospira*, of which there are a great many species, and which are responsible for other disease conditions in animals and man.

Equine periodic ophthalmia is characterized by periodic attacks of general inflammation of the eyeball, subsequent shrinking of same and finally blindness. It occurs under a variety of circumstances, usually in mature horses, and has in the past been more commonly seen when large numbers of horses have been congregated together, such as in the army. Odd sporadic cases do occur.

It had been observed that the disease was prone to occur in damp surroundings, on low-lying country and in dark ill-ventilated stables, and such conditions were held to be predisposing causes. The disease is much less common now throughout the world than it was formerly, due no doubt to decrease in the number of horses and improved sanitation. It is not a common disease in Australia.

Symptoms

The onset of the disease is sudden, and the first indication of the disease occurs when the horse is seen with half closed eyelids on one side, tears trickling down the face and evasion of bright light. The horse objects to handling of the eye and, when this is attempted, will keep the lids tightly closed. Careful examination will reveal inflammation of the conjunctiva and deeper parts of the eye, contraction of the pupil and perhaps some opacity of the cornea. This is usually associated with a slight rise in temperature and general depression. Other changes, including lack of lustre of the iris also occur in the eye. This initial period of inflammation may last from between two to ten days. This is followed by a gradual decline of all symptoms over a period of about three weeks, when, to a casual observer, the eye appears to be normal. Only very close examination and use of an ophthalmoscope will reveal remaining abnormalities. The characteristic recurrence of the disease occurs from three weeks to three months after the first attack. It may be in the same eye or in the other one. In the second attack, the symptoms are much the same as in the first but it takes longer for the eye to clear again. Each succeeding attack leaves its additional damage to the vital structures of the eye. After several attacks, the lens will show a number of fleecy lines running in towards the centre and soon the whole lens will become

G

a white and opaque mass and the animal will be blind. After an animal has had one or more attacks, the eyeball becomes perceptibly smaller than normal and the upper eyelid is wrinkled. The attacks vary greatly in severity in different cases, but the recurrence is quite distinctive and will lead to permanent blindness.

Treatment

This is essentially a matter for a veterinarian. A darkened stable or shed or even an eye-shade contributes to the animal's comfort during the period when it is very sensitive to light.

EYE—"DERMOID CYSTS"

A SO-CALLED dermoid "cyst" may develop in various situations in the body. The growth is a piece of skin which has become misplaced during the formation of the embryo before birth. This piece of embryonic skin continues to grow and produce hair wherever it is located in the body. In the eye, a dermoid "cyst", which should more correctly be referred to as a tumour, is commonly attached to the margin of the white tough outer membrane of the eyeball where it joins the cornea, and looks like a smooth wart. From its free surface grow hairs of variable length which cause irritation and excessive flow of tears, and may cause interference with vision and even ulceration of the cornea. The tumour can be removed under an anaesthetic by delicate surgery.

EYELIDS—ENTROPION

ENTROPION means a turning-in of the eyelid, usually the lower, in such a way that the lashes rub against the globe of the eye and cause irritation. The condition is more commonly seen in foals, when not infrequently the lids of both eyes are affected. In adult animals the condition may follow laceration and faulty healing of the eyelid. It may also occur as a sequel to severe conjunctivitis or an attack of periodic ophthalmia.

Symptoms

The irritation caused by the inverted lashes rubbing against the cornea may result in keratitis and loss of sight. The condition of entropion is recognized by a continuous closure of the eyelids with some suppuration and matting of the lashes.

Treatment

Some cases in foals will recover without surgical intervention and will respond simply to pulling out the lower lid and repeating the

84

procedure from time to time during the first few days of the foal's life.

Fortunately, quite a minor operation will cure the condition but this should be left to a veterinarian to perform under a local anaesthetic. It may only be necessary to suture the lid back into place, or remove an elliptical piece of skin from below the offending lid and suture the edges of the cut together. Either of these procedures, but particularly the latter, will cause sufficient contraction of the skin to pull back the lid and prevent it from curling inwards.

FALSE QUARTER

FALSE quarter is the term applied to that condition of the horn of the quarter of the foot in which, owing to disease or injury of the coronet, the wall has grown in a manner that is incomplete. It is seen more commonly on the fore feet and usually on the inner side, but does occur on the hind feet.

Causes

As already mentioned, false quarter can result from any disease of the foot that involves destruction of a portion of the coronary cushion, because it is from the papillae of this body that the horn tubules of the wall are secreted. Destruction of any part of it results in a corresponding loss of horn in that position. The disease of the foot which most commonly causes this is *quittor*. It may also result from a suppurating corn or from a severe tread or overreach.

Symptoms

The condition appears as a gap or shallow indentation, narrow or wide, in the thickness of the wall, with its length in the direction of the horn fibres. The condition is aggravated should there be a sandcrack in the quarter. On either side of the indentation an abnormal growth of horn occurs, which protrudes and stands above the level of the horn surrounding it. This might be regarded as a form of hypertrophy—abnormal increase in the size of a part—brought about by the increased stress imposed by the loss of substance in the region of the false quarter. So long as the sensitive structures of the foot are not exposed, the horse does not go lame. Sometimes, however, as a result of concussion, a fissure appears in the narrow veneer of horn that covers the sensitive structures in the indentation, aided perhaps by a sandcrack in the quarter. Infection then takes place, leading to inflammatory changes and pus formation, and the horse becomes lame. Many horses are not adversely affected for work by a false quarter which has not become infected, but the latter is always possible.

Treatment

The treatment of false quarter is exceedingly difficult because of destruction of the horn-secreting substance of the coronary cushion. The fissure in the wall usually remains, rendering the horse liable to occasional lameness and making that side of the hoof weak. Attention should be given to the coronary cushion injury and the horse appropriately shod to keep weight off the affected quarter.

FISTULA

A FISTULA is an abnormal tube-like passage which may exist in any part of the body. In horses, the term "fistula" has come to be commonly accepted as applicable only to such lesions when found on the withers. Poll evil is a fistula or sinus in the region of the poll and in no sense differs from *fistulous withers* other than in location. *Quittor* presents the characteristic tubular passages of a fistula and may, therefore, be considered and treated as a fistula of the foot. Fistulous passages may also be developed upon the sides of the face, through which saliva is discharged instead of flowing into the mouth, and they are called salivary fistulas. A dental fistula may arise from necrosis of the root of a tooth.

A fistula is sometimes noted at the umbilicus (navel) associated with hernia, and recto-vaginal fistulas have been developed in mares, following difficult parturition. A fistula of the oesophagus may occur as a result of misuse of a probang or stomach tube for the relief of choke.

Fistulous tracts persist whilst irritation occurs from some foreign body, necrotic bone, cartilage or other infective material, particularly when there is poor drainage from the part.

FISTULOUS WITHERS AND POLL EVIL

FISTULAS are particularly prone to develop at the withers or poll because the exposed position of these parts renders them liable to injury, but trauma or mechanical injury is not always necessary for infection to occur. Once infection is located in these areas it is inclined to extend further downwards, because of the fan-shaped way the muscles and tendons are arranged in these situations, thus allowing it to gravitate to the deeper-lying structures. It will be readily appreciated how quickly the bursa (the protective sheath covering the bones and even the bones themselves) together with the main ligament of the neck become involved, leading to *necrosis*. One of the most significant features of fistulous withers is that there are so many variations of the arrangement, size, location, and anatomical relations of these lesions. A knowledge of anatomy is necessary to fully appreciate why this is so.

Cause

Because the organisms of *Brucella abortus* and *Brucella suis*, the germs responsible for Brucellosis in cattle and pigs, have been cultured from cases of fistulous withers and poll evil, the possibility of infection of the horse with these germs has to be kept in mind as a cause of these conditions. Further, a microfilarial parasite (small thread-like worm) *Onchocerca reticulata* is not uncommonly found in the neck ligament of horses and has been held responsible for some cases. On the other hand, injury to the parts and subsequent infection with pus-producing and other organisms is a more common cause. Among the more common predisposing causes of fistulous withers are bad fitting collars or saddles; direct injury from blows or stallion bites, and rolling upon rough or sharp stones. Saddle horses that are very low in the withers permit the saddle to ride forward and

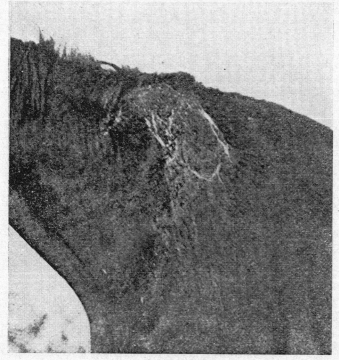

Fig. 46 Fistulous wither of long standing. There is considerable inflammation, with hair, skin and underlying tissues destroyed.

(United States Department of Agriculture)

87

bruise the parts, and are prone to be affected with fistulous withers. *Poll evil* may follow chafing by a halter, headstall or heavy bridle, blows from the butt end of a whip, the horse striking its head against a beam, low stable doors and so on.

Following the initial injury, infection occurs leading to inflammatory swelling and often to abscess formation below the skin, which, if not quickly and properly treated, may become fistulous. This results from pus seeping between the muscles and escaping only when pressure forces it to the surface, and it bursts through the skin.

Should the fistulous wither or poll evil be caused by *Brucella abortus* infection, the discharges can contaminate the pasture, so that a horse affected with these conditions can be the means of transmitting Brucellosis to cattle or other horses grazing over such pasture.

Symptoms

The symptoms vary according to the progress of the fistula. When the wither is affected, the horse may at first show some soreness or stiffness of the front legs. In a day or two a swelling commonly occurs on one or both sides of the wither, which is usually hot and painful. The stiffness of the limbs may disappear at this time and the heat and soreness of the swelling may become less noticeable, although it continues to enlarge. Several months may elapse before the swelling bursts at some point and discharges. The discharge may cease and the opening may apparently heal, only to break out again later.

Poll evil may be first indicated by the animal becoming sensitive to the application of the bridle or to a grooming brush. The disease in its early stages may be recognized as a soft fluctuating swelling on one or both sides of the mid-line of the poll surrounded by inflammatory swelling, and stiffness of the neck. Later the inflammation of the surrounding tissues may disappear, leaving a prominent tumour-like swelling. Subsequently this swelling bursts and discharges and, as in the case of fistulous withers, heals up temporarily and discharges again.

Treatment

The treatment of fistula of the withers or fistula of the poll (poll evil) is determined by the changes that have occurred in the affected structures. It is essentially a matter for a qualified veterinary surgeon. In the earliest stages of the diseases, when there is soreness, perhaps enlarged lymphatic vessels, and only slight swelling, the trouble might be checked by hot fomentations, massage, and the application of tincture of iodine or iodine ointment daily. In other cases where the swelling is simply due to a sterile distension of the synovial sac

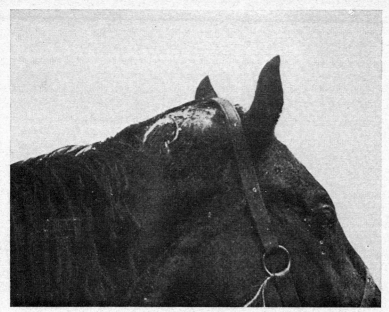

Fig. 47   Poll Evil.
(United States Department of Agriculture)

covering the bones, the condition may respond to the daily scrubbing in of tincture of iodine with a small brush, or better still to the intravenous injection of sodium iodide, which would necessarily have to be carried out by a veterinarian. Once the swelling has burst and is discharging pus, treatment is outside the province of the horse-owner. Home treatments with strong caustic drugs and arsenic, and the use of setons are seldom successful and usually involve much suffering to the horse. From the foregoing description of the two disease conditions, it will be appreciated that surgical intervention is the only way of arranging for proper drainage and the removal of necrotic material which is causing the trouble. Combined with surgery, the veterinarian will adopt antibiotic and other forms of treatment in an attempt to cure these very troublesome conditions. Sometimes an extended daily course of antibiotic treatment given by or under the supervision of a veterinarian will effect a cure, and then only if there is not extensive involvement of the bone and ligaments.

FLIES

THE COMMON house-fly (*Musca domestica*), the bush-fly (*Musca vetustissima*) and the stable-fly (*Stomoxys calcitrans*) are the main

89

flies which worry horses in Australia. March-flies (*Tabanus spp.*) also worry horses and inflict a severe bite. All these flies can carry disease. Reference has already been made (see *Eye—Habronemic Conjunctivitis*) to the fact that house-flies, bush-flies and stable-flies act as intermediate hosts of certain species of stomach worms of the genus *Habronema*. The larvae of these worms are carried by flies into the eyes and onto abrasions on the body of the horse and give rise to *habronemic conjunctivitis* and a skin condition known as "summer sores". It is suggested that swamp cancer of horses may have a similar origin.

Bush-flies, when feeding on the secretions of the mouth, eyes, ears, nose and around the vulva, as they commonly do in great numbers, cause considerable irritation to the animal. The flesh around these areas is indented and the skin raised, due, it is presumed, to the secretion of digestive juices by the flies.

Stable- and March-flies annoy horses and the females of certain species of the latter suck blood.

The buffalo-fly, which is normally associated with cattle and buffaloes, will attack horses but only when they are with cattle. This fly can only live where its bovine host exists, as it breeds in the freshly dropped dung.

Control

The most effective method of controlling house-flies and stable-flies is by the regular and thorough collection of manure, and its treatment or disposal so that flies cannot breed in it. Manure is most attractive to flies during the first three to five days. Flies will not breed in dry dung and desiccation kills the eggs. If practicable, dung should be collected and spread as soon as possible over pasture where it will quickly dry out. Alternatively, dung should be tightly packed, and every four days the heap should be raked and the old dung placed on top of the fresh dung. This raises the temperature of the dung heap and the fly eggs are destroyed. Fly-proof pits can be used, or the dung heap sprayed with one of the organic phosphorus preparations to destroy the emerging flies. It is much more difficult to control bush- and March-flies by the above methods as their breeding places are very extensive. Various sprays may be used to kill the adult flies on the horse, which will at least afford temporary relief to the animal. The hair on the tail, mane and forelock should not be interfered with, and a leather fly veil attached to a headstall will assist in protecting the eyes. When severe waves of bush-flies occur, it is a common practice in the country to light smudge fires around which horses will congregate to get smoke protection from the flies.

FOAL—REARING OF ORPHAN

WHEN a mare dies or has no milk, it becomes necessary to raise the foal by hand. Sometimes it is possible to arrange for another recently-foaled mare to take the foal in addition to her own, or to put the foal on to a recently calved cow of a large breed, such as a Friesian or Shorthorn. Usually it is necessary to rear the foal on fresh cow's or goat's milk diluted with one-third the quantity of warm, boiled water and sweetened with one ounce of sugar to the quart of milk mixture. This milk mixture is similar to the milk of the mare which has low butter fat and high sugar content. One to two teaspoonfuls of vitamin A standardized cod liver oil should be added to each quart of milk and water mixture for the first ten days. Lactose or milk sugar is the best kind of sugar to use and is available from any chemist. Glucose can also be used. The milk mixture should be warmed to blood heat and the foal given ½ a pint every two hours at the beginning.

After a few days, if the foal is doing well, the quantities of milk and the intervals between feeds can be increased until the foal is getting 4 pints of milk three times a day when a month old. More milk may be given if the foal seems to need it, but overfeeding should be avoided. The sugar may be reduced at three weeks of age and discontinued at one month. At six to eight weeks, skim milk may be gradually substituted for whole milk. By three months, the foal may be given all the milk it can drink, which may be up to two gallons a day. It should, of course, have access to clean drinking water. A bottle with a large rubber teat can be used to feed the very young foal but it should be encouraged to drink from an open vessel as soon as possible. Scrupulous cleanliness must be observed with the bottle and teat, which should be sterilized after use and kept covered with a clean cloth until used again. All vessels used to hold milk must be rinsed with cold water immediately after use and then scalded and kept covered.

The foal will begin to nibble grass at about three weeks. Feeding of a dry meal or crushed oats may be commenced at four weeks. Three parts of crushed oats to one part of bran makes a suitable concentrate mixture. Some prime quality lucerne hay should be available to the foal and, if there is a shortage of green grass, some greenstuff should be fed. At about two months the foal will be eating a considerable quantity of crushed oats and hay, especially if the grazing is poor. Lucerne hay is a valuable source of calcium (lime) and it is recommended that some be fed, even if the foal is running on good grass pasture. If lucerne hay is not fed regularly, one per cent of finely ground limestone should be added to the concentrate mixture. Skim milk feeding should continue until the foal is five to six months old or even a little longer if the milk is available, when the foal may be weaned. At least one feed of crushed oats should be given daily until the end of the first year.

An orphan foal should be suitably housed and protected from cold winds and rain. The shed should be kept clean and any bedding, such as straw, frequently changed. If possible, a companion animal should be kept with the foal. A quiet old pony is best, but a quiet calf, sheep or goat will help. This prevents the foal from being lonely, and it learns to eat, seek shelter, and fend for itself more rapidly.

Young foals are subject to a number of diseases which are discussed elsewhere. Within the first twelve hours of life, a foal is likely to be constipated, especially if it has not sucked the mother and obtained the colostrum. The constipated condition is due to retention of the meconium (the first dung discharges of the new-born). A home method of correcting this is to give the foal an enema of 1 part of glycerine in 5 parts of warm water, using an ordinary human enema syringe, after lubricating the nozzle with white petroleum jelly. It will frequently be necessary to repeat the enema. Four ounces of liquid paraffin should also be given, preferably with a stomach tube but otherwise very carefully as a drench. Diarrhoea may occur, often as a result of incorrect feeding or overfeeding, and is usually complicated by bacterial infection of the bowels.

The services of a veterinary surgeon should be obtained, so that appropriate sulphonamide or antibiotic treatment can be carried out without delay. Bacterial infection can be largely avoided by strict attention to hygiene and care with feeding bottles and utensils. For details of treatment see *Diarrhoea*.

FOUNDER (Laminitis)

THE CORRECT name for founder is laminitis and this gives a clue to the nature of the disease. It is an inflammation of the sensitive laminae and other vascular structures of the foot. The sensitive laminae form the junction between the hard insensitive hoof and the underlying soft sensitive structures. They consist of thin fleshy ridges or plates running parallel with each other, which fit into corresponding depressions on the inner surface of the horny wall and sole of the foot. Inflammation of the sensitive laminae leads to an increase in the volume of blood within the horny box of the hoof which, together with stagnation of venous blood, causes great pain and foot-soreness. If this congestion is not speedily relieved, serious consequences commonly result.

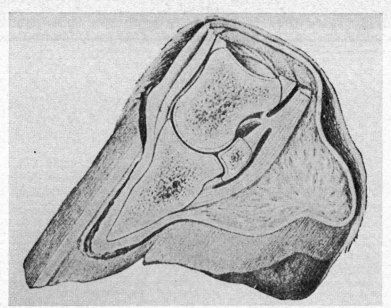

Fig. 48 Longitudinal Section of a Foot with Laminitis of eight days'
standing.
(*From Diseases of the Horse's Foot. H. Carlton Reeks. Bailliere, Tindall & Cox*)

a

b

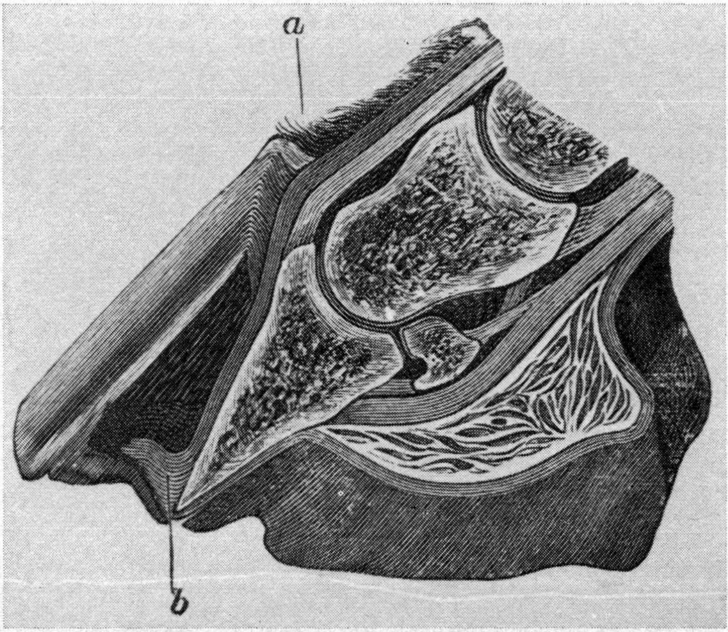

Fig. 49 Longitudinal Section of a Foot with Laminitis of fourteen days'
standing.
(*From Diseases of the Horse's Foot. H. Carlton Reeks. Bailliere, Tindall & Cox*)

Causes

The causes and predisposing causes of the disease are of great variety and some horses are more prone to contract the disease than others. The following are some of the causes of laminitis: sudden changes of food, especially engorgement on wheat and other grains to which the horse is unaccustomed; severe work after a period of idleness, or severe work at fast pace on hard ground; lack of exercise, as when horses are sent on long sea voyages, or when they are kept in stalls for long periods and do not lie down; overweight, especially if associated with lack of exercise, and commonly seen in fat ponies at grass; metritis (inflammation of the womb) after foaling; exhaustion; flat-footedness, and as a complication of pneumonia. Horses which are lame in one foot or leg and favour this limb, may develop laminitis in the foot of the opposite leg.

Symptoms

Laminitis more frequently affects the fore than the hind feet. The symptoms, which usually occur suddenly, vary according to whether the animal is affected in one or more feet. The most marked symptom is lameness, the animal being unwilling to move. When the fore feet are affected, the body is thrown backwards, the horse putting the weight on the hind legs, which are placed well forward under the belly. The forelegs are extended well in front. If the hind feet only are involved, all four legs are held under the body to relieve the hind feet of as much weight as possible. When all feet are affected, the horse stands with the back arched and the hind legs drawn forward under the body to take most of the weight on the heels. If forced to move, the animal walks on its heels, lifting the feet quickly in a characteristic crouching manner. In acute cases, the temperature is raised, the breathing is heavy and hurried, the pulse rate is increased and the animal may break out in a sweat.

Examination of the feet at this stage will reveal nothing abnormal except that the hooves of the affected feet will feel hotter than normal, and pressure with the thumbs, or light tapping with a hammer, may be resented because of pain. The artery at the back of the fetlock throbs beneath the finger. In most cases of laminitis the horse remains standing, but in some cases it lies down on its side with the legs extended.

Treatment

Recovery from this disease depends on early diagnosis and prompt treatment before permanent injury takes place. Professional assistance should be sought if possible. A quick-acting purgative and the injection of antihistamine drugs are indicated. A very important part of reatment which should be commenced without delay, and even efore arrival of the veterinarian, is cold applications to the feet fter removal of the shoes. It may be carried out by standing the orse in a dam or creek, or in a foot-bath dug in the yard or paddock nd filled with water. The horse should be tied to a rail or held in uch a way as to compel him to keep the affected feet in the water. Alternatively, the feet may be placed in buckets of very cold water, sing ice if available, for an hour at a time, three or four times a day. orced exercise by a short slow walk for ten minutes every hour or the first 48 hours is also recommended, provided the pain is not o severe.

Bleeding from the jugular vein may be beneficial but this is a natter which should be decided by the veterinarian. In any case, he as drugs at his disposal which will have the same effect. The horse hould be given a laxative diet of bran mashes and green grass, if vailable.

If treatment as outlined above is begun early, the acute cases sually subside within five or six days. The animal should not be eturned to work for at least three weeks after recovery.

CHRONIC LAMINITIS

Chronic laminitis results when the acute disease progresses to roduce deformity of the foot. The sole drops, rings develop on the oof running parallel with the coronet and the hoof may become nisshapen. A cure of this condition is extremely difficult, and the orse is usually rendered unfit for ordinary work. By judicious paring f the foot and with special shoeing, a horse may have some degree f usefulness.

FRACTURES

ALL the bones of the body are subject to fractures but in the horse nost fractures are of the bones of the limbs. Other fractures which re not so common involve the face, the lower jaw, the ribs, cervical ertebrae and the pelvic bones. Different terms are given to the arious types of fractures, the more common ones being *greenstick r incomplete fracture*, where only part of the bone is broken or the one cracks or splits; *simple fracture*, when the bone is broken ight through but the soft parts have received no injury and there is o external wound; *compound fracture*, when one broken end of a one causes an external wound; *comminuted fracture*, when the bone as been broken in several places and shattered; *impacted fracture*, when one broken end of a bone is driven in to the other broken end.

Causes

Apart from certain predisposing causes such as age, fragility of th
bones due to disease, slippery conditions of roads and tracks, mos
fractures in horses are caused by direct violence, such as kicks, falls
errors in judgement during jumping, collisions, casting for operations
or from sudden or excessive muscular contractions as may occur i
galloping or jumping, or by struggling when cast for operation.

Symptoms

Usually fractures are easily diagnosed because the part is rendere
useless, crepitation—grating of fractured bones—can be heard or fe
when manipulated, and there is unnatural mobility and deformity
Sometimes, however, such as in the case of a fractured pelvis or spl
pastern bone, these symptoms are not observed, and, although the
may be revealed by careful manipulation, an X-ray is often necessary

Treatment

Skilled veterinary attention is required for the treatment of mos
fractures in the horse but the type of animal, the use to which it i
put, the nature of the fracture and economic considerations influenc
the decision as to whether treatment is justified. The reason wh
veterinary surgeons commonly recommend the destruction of a hors
with a broken leg is an economic one, because it is uneconomic t
put a horse in a sling for a long period and, in spite of the bes
treatment, to have a horse left lame. Treatment may be justified fc
sentimental reasons or the value of the animal for breeding purposes

Bones of the horse heal quite well if the broken parts can be kep
in apposition—a much more difficult matter than in the case of sma
animals. After reduction of the fracture, splints, plaster of pari
bandages and other supports may be used for this purpose and bone
may be plated or pinned surgically. The difficulty is to keep th
patient in a state of rest and quietness, hence the difficulty of gettin
complete recoveries. As long bones have a tendency to shorten whei
uniting, a break of the leg commonly leaves a horse slightly lame.

In the case of incomplete or greenstick fractures in foals wher
there is no displacement, complete recovery may occur if the foa
can be kept quiet in a loose-box or shed.

FROG—DISEASES OF

See *Canker, Thrush*

THE FROG is intended to act as a cushion to take the first weight o
the limb. A healthy frog does not bruise, and the best way of bringin
a diseased one back to health is to lower the heels and give it groun

pressure. Ragged edges of the frog which harbour dirt may be trimmed off, but no cutting away of the healthy frog should be allowed. Attention to stable hygiene and cleanliness of the part are essential in preventing diseases of the frog.

GASTRO-ENTERITIS

GASTRITIS signifies an inflammation of the stomach and *enteritis* an inflammation of the intestines. The two conditions commonly occur together, when the disease is referred to as gastro-enteritis.

Causes

The diseased conditions may be caused by irritant food, mouldy or decayed food, internal parasites and chemical poisons. They also occur in certain acute infectious diseases such as anthrax, and may follow long-continued obstruction of the bowels (obstruction colic) or displacement of the bowels.

Symptoms

The symptoms vary to some extent with the cause and depend on the chief location, extent and severity of the inflammation. The animal shows colicky pains; develops a fever; pulse and respiration become rapid; the mucous membranes of the eyes become red, and the mouth is hot and dry. Pressure on the abdomen may cause pain; legs are cold. Sometimes small hard pellets of dung are passed, covered with slime and evil-smelling. The urine may be scanty and highly coloured.

Treatment

Prompt professional assistance is necessary for the treatment of these severe conditions in horses, and such treatment will depend on the nature of the causative agent. Home treatment is seldom successful. If the inflammation is associated with irritant or damaged food, 2 to 3 pints of liquid paraffin should be given by stomach tube or as a drench. Good nursing may save an animal. Frequent hot fomentations to the body with blankets, and warm enemas are useful. A liquid diet is indicated, and oatmeal gruel, hay tea or rice water should be given for the first twenty-four hours. Later, small light feeds, such as freshly-prepared bran mashes, may be fed. The horse must be kept warm by rugging and the legs rubbed and bandaged with woollen or Newmarket bandages. If the horse is in great pain, 1 oz. of chloral hydrate may be given in one and a half pints of milk as a drench. Chlorodyne or tincture of opium may be of value in some cases. If the condition is due to poisoning, the appropriate antidote will be necessary.

GIRTH GALLS

A GALL is an excoriation (erosion) of the skin and commonly results from excessive pressure or friction imposed on a horse's body by the saddle, the girth and harness generally, and is frequently associated with the condition or shape of the animal. Condition certainly plays an important part in the causation of girth galls, as horses in soft condition gall much more readily than horses in hard condition. Hard, dirty girths contribute to galling, but under ordinary conditions it is not so much the hardness of the girth that causes the gall, but rather its movement forward so that the edge of the girth is dragged forward behind the elbow. The shape of the brisket around which the girth fits, and the general conformation of the chest contribute to this. It can sometimes be overcome by using a split leather girth (not generally recommended) which catches not only the edge of the brisket, but also the skin. A girth should be kept fairly tight to ensure that it moves as little as possible. In this connection it should be remembered that a saddle is never girthed to a back as tightly as it seems, because when the rider's weight is in the saddle, the girth at once becomes slacker. Some horses learn the trick of keeping their chests distended with air when they are being girthed up. If necessary, such horses should have their girths tightened again by someone after the rider is in the saddle.

When, owing to malformation of the horse, the girth persists in slipping forward, it can be held back by means of a surcingle and a strap. The surcingle is placed under the seat towards the rear arch of the saddle, and passed obliquely under the belly and buckled. A strap is then applied along the underline from girth to surcingle which should be about a foot to the rear of the girth. If the horse already has a girth gall, the saddle girth can be drawn back as far as is considered necessary to avoid the injured surface, and then drawn tight. The strap is adjusted and then the surcingle tightened, but only sufficiently to prevent it from being drawn forward. With such a contrivance, the girth does not slip forward, galling is prevented and it is possible to work a horse with a simple girth gall.

When girth galls occur because of soft condition, a piece of sheepskin or soft rubber tubing placed around the girth will prevent galling until the horse improves in condition.

Treatment for simple girth gall

Wash the excoriated skin with warm water and soap; allow to dry; dab on white lotion (zinc sulphate 1 oz., lead acetate 1 oz., water 1 pint) several times a day, or apply a solution of triple dyes, obtainable from any chemist. Neglected galls which have become infected will require veterinary attention.

GREASE—GREASY HEEL

THE SCIENTIFIC name for grease or greasy heel is *seborrhoea*, which means an abnormal secretion of the sebaceous or oil glands. It is accompanied by deep-seated inflammation of the skin at the rear surfaces of the pastern and fetlock and is really a chronic dermatitis. The specific cause is unknown, but the condition is usually seen in heavy horses with coarse thick legs, when such horses are kept in damp, dirty stables or are long subjected to mud and filth without proper grooming. It can, however, occur in any type of horse and is sometimes seen in horses with clean legs kept under hygienic conditions.

Symptoms

The early symptoms are swelling and redness of the skin, with some itching. Later there is increased secretion from the sebaceous glands in the affected area, over which the hair stands erect, the individual hairs being glued together by the oily secretion. The skin, which is at first moist and sensitive, tends to become thickened and later fungoid masses commonly referred to as "grapes" may be found, and the part enlarges considerably. Secondary bacterial infection occurs, leading to necrosis and ulceration. There is an offensive odour. The infection may spread to the frog and even undermine the sole of the foot. The hind legs are most commonly affected but the condition is seen in the forelegs. Lameness may or may not be present.

Treatment

Early cases of the disease, when only the superficial layers of the skin are involved, will respond to local treatment. When the condition is advanced, the prognosis is not so hopeful. The hair should be clipped closely over the affected areas, and the part then cleansed with good quality soap and water, rubbing the soap in gently for some time. Wipe off any fungoid or greasy material. When thoroughly dry, apply a mild astringent lotion, such as white lotion (see *Girth Galls*) repeatedly, but keep the part soft with benzoated zinc oxide ointment or zinc cream. Bluestone solution (1 oz. bluestone to a pint of water) may be used as an early application. Good results have been reported following repeated dusting of the affected areas, after thorough washing and drying, with a sulphonamide dusting powder. Advanced cases of the disease will require attention by a veterinarian.

Preventive measures for greasy heels include refraining from unnecessary washing of the legs and feet and, when this is unavoidable, thorough drying of the legs. Clipping the legs for appearance' sake should be avoided. Oiling behind the pastern and fetlock in prolonged wet weather, and attention to hygiene are the most effective ways to prevent occurrence of the condition.

HEART DISEASES

STRUCTURAL heart diseases are rare in horses but functional troubles are not uncommon. The causes are various and are beyond the scope of a layman to diagnose.

Symptoms

Weakness, distress on exertion, panting, irregular pulse, wave passing up the jugular vein, blueness of lips and eyelids, thumping of heart behind elbow and sudden death.

Treatment

Professional attention is necessary.

HEATSTROKE—HEAT EXHAUSTION— SUNSTROKE

THE CONDITIONS known as heatstroke, heat exhaustion and sunstroke are due to severe brain disturbance and upset of the heat-regulating mechanism of the body. In general, they result from high environmental temperature, high humidity and sometimes inadequate ventilation. Heatstroke and heat exhaustion occur in excessively hot humid weather when horses are crowded together in yards or cattle trucks, or are forced to work hard in such weather. Sunstroke is caused when animals are unable to find shade and are exposed to direct rays of the sun, and more particularly, if they are worked continuously in the sun during very hot weather. Lack of water is an important contributing factor.

Symptoms

The symptoms of heatstroke, heat exhaustion and sunstroke, which develop suddenly, are, with minor variations, very similar. The horse is usually very distressed, the breathing is hurried, the temperature very high, the nostrils are dilated and highly reddened, the pulse is rapid and weak, usually sweating is checked, the pupils of the eyes are dilated, and the horse staggers and falls to the ground partially or totally unconscious. Whilst on the ground, if not fully unconscious, he may struggle and attempt to get up but be unable to do so. Muscular spasms or convulsions may be shown. Death occurs quickly in some cases but less severe ones recover, especially if treatment can be carried out promptly.

100

Treatment

The horse should be moved to a cool and shady spot, the head and neck freely douched with cold water and fanned. Ice packs should be applied to the top and sides of the head and along the jugular furrow. If possible, the whole body, especially the spine, should be hosed, particularly in the case of heatstroke, in an attempt to reduce the body temperature, and this should be repeated at intervals so that the temperature drops gradually. Cold water should be available to the animal to drink immediately he is able to do so. Good nursing, a light diet and a lengthy spell from work are necessary for full recovery. Veterinary surgeons administer various stimulants subcutaneously and supplement the cold applications by intravenous injections of saline and other solutions.

HEELS—DISEASES OF

See *Cracked Heels, Grease—Greasy Heel*

HERNIA (Rupture)

A HERNIA is a protrusion of any organ or part of an organ through the containing wall of its cavity, beyond its normal confines. The term is usually applied to the abdominal cavity, but hernias occur elsewhere in the body.

Abdominal hernias, or ruptures, may be classified as *reducible*, when the protruding structures can be readily pushed back into the abdominal cavity through the hernial ring; *irreducible*, when the structures have become adherent to the surroundings, or have become enlarged after emerging, or for other reasons cannot be pushed back; *strangulated*, when the circulation of the blood to the herniated bowel is cut off by the margin of the opening through which the loop of bowel has passed, thereby causing congestion, swelling and inflammation which, if not promptly relieved, leads to gangrene of the part and death of the animal.

According to their situation, abdominal hernias are described as umbilical, scrotal, inguinal, and ventral, and may be congenital or acquired.

UMBILICAL HERNIA

This form of hernia commonly occurs in foals and results from imperfect closure of the umbilicus, which is the opening through which the umbilical cord passes before birth. A loop of bowel or omentum (caul) passes through this opening, either at birth or subsequently, as a result of strain and weakness of the muscle, and lies just beneath the skin. Constipation or diarrhoea may lead to

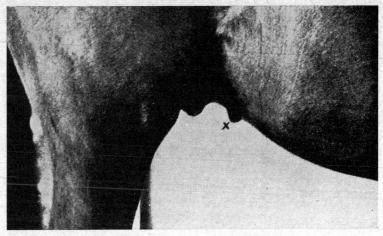

Fig. 50 Umbilical Hernia or Rupture at X.
(*United States Department of Agriculture*)

umbilical hernia in the early life of the foal. The soft swelling can usually be pushed back easily with the fingers, especially if the animal is placed on its back. There is no pain and the health of the foal is not affected.

Most of these hernias disappear spontaneously without any form of treatment, favoured by the small size of the rupture, absence of adhesions, youth of the animal and growth of the abdomen. As the abdomen expands in diameter, the protruding portion of the intestine and omentum are drawn gradually into the abdominal cavity. This may take twelve months. Bearing this in mind, hasty action should not be taken to rectify umbilical hernias in foals, and provided they do not enlarge or become hot and painful, they are best left alone. Should any of these complications appear, professional assistance should be sought, as an operation is then frequently necessary to correct the hernia and prevent strangulation. Umbilical hernias which occur later in life require surgical attention.

SCROTAL AND INGUINAL HERNIAS

These forms of hernia are also fairly common in foals as congenital conditions. The foal is born with an enlarged scrotum ("purse"), caused by a piece of omentum or bowel having descended through the inguinal canal into the scrotum.

An inguinal hernia is one in which the piece of omentum or bowel descends, but remains in the inguinal canal. It is not so evident as a scrotal hernia. Both these forms of hernia are due to the abdominal

102

end of the canal being unusually large. Again, as in the case of umbilical hernia, these conditions rectify themselves over a period of twelve months or less provided there are no complications. In those cases where pain is shown or strangulation appears to be imminent, an immediate operation is necessary. Acquired scrotal and inguinal hernias in older animals, caused as a result of strain or over-exertion, can only be reduced by operation.

VENTRAL HERNIA

This is a hernia which mostly occurs as a result of some injury to the abdominal wall, which is weakened and allows portion of the bowel or omentum to pass through an artificial opening. Congenital perforations of the walls of the abdomen of the foal do sometimes occur, but are rare. An injury, such as a kick from another horse, a fall upon a stump or large stone, or even a kick from a man's boot, are common causative factors. These hernias vary greatly in size depending on the dimensions of the aperture, and may occur anywhere on the dependent parts of the abdomen. Treatment is by operation under a general anaesthetic.

HOCK—DISEASES OF

HOCK SPRAIN

A sprain of the hock may give rise to symptoms similar to those of bone spavin, of which it may be the forerunner: it involves the tendons and other structures of the hock. It is a fairly common condition, being a result of over-extension of the joint as may occur in jumping, or slipping on a wet smooth surface. Depending on the extent of the injury, hock sprain may be slight or very severe. Following a severe sprain, there may be haemorrhage from the torn structures leading to considerable swelling of the joint. It is difficult to estimate the damage done by such a severe sprain because inflammation may extend to the joint causing a synovitis and possibly also arthritis and ostitis. When the whole hock is involved, the condition is commonly referred to as *sprung hock*. The symptoms are marked lameness, and swelling around the area with heat and tenderness on pressure. The horse rests the leg and may be unable to lie down. Treatment involves rest, hot and cold fomentations, poultices, followed by massage and the use of stimulating liniments. If the condition becomes chronic, blistering and other forms of joint treatment by a veterinarian will be necessary.

See *Capped Hock, Curb, Spavin, Thoroughpin*

103

HOOF—DISEASES OF

WHILST the hoof is the hard horny casing of the foot, it is so intimately related to the other structures of the foot that it is common to consider hoof diseases and foot diseases together. Books have been written on diseases of the horse's foot, including the hoof, and when one considers the importance of a horse having four good feet this is not surprising. The scope of this book does not permit a detailed description of the anatomy and physiology of the horse's foot, but the following brief discussion will help to explain a number of troubles attributable directly or indirectly to improper management or to faulty conformation.

The hoof of the horse and of other solipeds may well be compared with the human fingernail except that it completely encases the digit. The wall of the hoof consists of more or less dense, fibrous, horny material derived from the coronary band (the spongy tissue just above the hoof at its junction with the skin). Within this horny box are bones, tendons, ligaments, nerves and an intricate network of blood vessels. The hoof wall and sole are attached to the underlying structures by means of so-called sensitive and insensitive laminae (see under *Founder*). These consist of small leaf-like structures which are closely united in dovetailed fashion. Although the hoof would appear to be unyielding, it expands and contracts in waves when the animal moves on it, particularly at the heels and coronary cushion. Even the sole of the foot, which is superimposed over a padlike structure known as the plantar cushion, flattens out when weight is borne. The so-called lateral cartilages (referred to under *Sidebones*) play an important part in this normal expansion and contraction. The nutriment for the structures of the foot is received from the blood, the flow of which is largely controlled by the expansion and contraction of the parts referred to above. The hoof wall grows at the rate of about a quarter of an inch a month, being pushed down from the coronet regularly all around the foot. Growth is favoured by moisture, good nutrition and general health, as well as by exercise. The unshod hoof grows more rapidly than one with shoes.

The white line at the junction of the wall with the sole marks the point of union between the horny leaves of the sole and those of the wall. In shoeing, the nails are driven through the hoof at a point just outside this line. The sole is marked by a deep V-shaped cleft, outlined on each side by the bars, which are a continuation of the wall. The triangular-shaped horny structure within the lines of the V formed by the bars is known as the frog. The entire sole of the hoof, as well as the walls, cover highly sensitive tissue richly supplied with nerves and blood vessels.

The conformation of the ideal foot, that is the general form, outline and arrangement of parts, varies somewhat with the type of animal and even with the breed. Broadly, the well-shaped hoof is roughly like a cone from above downward. The print made by the hoof is generally oval, being slightly greater in length than in width. The walls of the hoof slope gradually and evenly outward from above and are free from deep grooves or bulges. The substance of the normal hoof is dense and firm but not brittle, and it has a distinctive natural gloss, the result of a varnish-like substance called periople, which lessens the evaporation of the moisture normally present in the horn. The bars are well defined, strong and widely spaced. There is no compressed narrowing of the foot at the heel, and the frog is clean and well formed. The feet should be centred on a perpendicular line from the point of the buttocks through the hock and fetlock in the hind leg and from the shoulder through the knee and fetlock in the front leg. Viewed from the side, the axis through the fetlock, pastern, and hoof should consist of a straight, unbroken line forming an angle of about 34° with the base of the foot. The hoof at the heel should generally be approximately one-third as long as in front. The foot of the donkey or mule is considerably smaller and rounder than the foot of the horse.

CONTRACTED HEELS

A condition not uncommonly seen affecting the heels and quarters, particularly of the feet of light horses, is that of contracted heels or "hoofbound". Horses which have been improperly shod so that the frog does not receive normal ground pressure are apt to be affected with contracted feet, particularly at the heels. Flat feet and low weak heels also predispose to this condition. Excessive use of the rasp from heel to toe, so that too much horn is removed from the heel and bars, may also be a factor in causing the condition. Lameness may occur especially at speed or after hard work.

Contracted heels of long standing may be difficult to rectify, and any treatment of the hoof is a slow process, extending over six months or more. If the animal can be allowed to go barefooted, this permits of natural pressure on the frog, and spreading of the heels will follow. If shoeing is necessary, the toe of the foot should be kept short and the bars and frog left alone as much as possible. Several grooves, parallel to the coronet and half an inch apart, may be cut into the quarters with a saw, starting three-quarters of an inch below the hairline and extending from the heel halfway to the toe. This operation must be repeated as the quarters grow out until the heels and quarters are normally expanded. Hoof ointments, containing such substances as turpentine, tar and wax in an oily or fatty base, should be used to assist in softening the horn. Special shoes, having as their object the spreading of the heels, are also useful.

BRITTLE HOOVES

As the name indicates, an abnormally dry state of the horn may develop as a result of which the hoof chips and cracks easily. Brittle hooves tend to predispose to contracted heels and lead to difficulties in shoeing. Long-continued dryness or stabling on hard dry floors is conducive to the trouble, as is also the horse's diet (lack of green feed). Brittle hooves require very careful shoeing to ensure that the bearing surface is as level as possible. Only thin nails should be used, placed in the strongest parts of the hoof wall. A hoof ointment of the type referred to under *Contracted Heels* should be used. Castor oil and lanoline make useful hoof dressings for this condition. Attention should be paid to the diet of the horse and, if natural grazing is not available, cut green feed should be fed. Should this not be possible, stabilized vitamin A should be fed in the concentrate ration.

See *Canker*, *Corns*, *False Quarter*, *Founder (laminitis)*, *Navicular Disease*, *Ringbone*, *Sand Crack*, *Seedy Toe*, *Sidebones*, *Shoeing Pricks*, *Thrush* and *Wounds*

INDIGESTION (Dyspepsia)

INDIGESTION is synonymous with dyspepsia and covers imperfect digestion and discomfort not only in the stomach but also elsewhere in the intestinal tract.

Causes

The causes of indigestion are numerous, but nearly all are the result of errors in feeding. Anything that irritates the stomach and intestines may cause the disease. Food to which the horse is unaccustomed, sudden changes of diet, imperfectly cured hay or chaff, or damaged foods are all likely causes. Over-filling of the stomach, hard work after a full feed, imperfect chewing due to bad teeth, cooked foods, injudicious use of medicines, internal parasites, wind-sucking and crib-biting are some of the other causes.

Symptoms

Loss of condition; irregular appetite; depraved appetite (disposition to eat unusual substances, such as wood, dung and soiled bedding); irregular bowel action, the dung being loose and bad-smelling or sometimes hard and dry; grain passed whole. There may be colicky pains and sometimes swelling of the abdomen and laboured breathing; the horse yawns, draws chin to chest and may lean against the wall of the stable. If the condition persists, the coat becomes harsh and dry.

Treatment

Attention to feeding and avoidance of the causes listed are more important than medicines. A laxative drench, such as 8 oz. of *Epsom* or *Glauber's* salts and 4 oz. of sodium bicarbonate (baking soda) in a pint of water, might be given to advantage. If the condition is suspected to be due to internal parasitic infection, appropriate treatment should be carried out. If there is a persistent tendency to flatulence, 2 oz. of sodium bicarbonate may be mixed in the daily allowance of feed. An ounce of salt should be given daily in the feed, or salt made readily available to the horse, preferably as rock-salt. The following old-time powder mixture has much to recommend it: Glauber's salts 2 lb., common salt 1 lb., baking soda 1 lb.—mix well together and put a tablespoonful in each feed.

"INFLUENZA"—EQUINE

THE DISEASE known as equine influenza, commonly referred to as "pink-eye" and considered to be due to a virus, complicated by secondary bacterial infection, has been the subject of intensive research over the last fifteen years. This has resulted in the identification of three specific viral diseases having symptoms which conform to the standard description of equine influenza. These three viral diseases are equine viral rhinopneumonitis, equine viral arteritis and a febrile respiratory catarrh caused by a myxovirus having properties of the A-type influenza viruses.

The disease formerly known as equine influenza, which occurred in severe epidemics in Australia in the 'eighties and at the turn of the present century, appears to have disappeared and no epizootics of this disease have occurred since 1912. This is supported by the fact that the disease did not appear in remount depots in Australia, nor on transports from Australia during the 1914-18 War, nor in horses mobilized during the earlier years of the Second World War.

As yet, diseases caused by the rhinopneumonitis virus and the arteritis virus do not appear to have assumed great importance in Australia. Both of these, in addition to causing symptoms of influenza, also cause abortion in mares.

107

Symptoms

The general symptoms of equine viral respiratory diseases (influenza) are those of high fever, marked depression, inflammation of the upper respiratory tract and sometimes of the intestines, and severe reddening of the mucous membranes of the eyes (hence the common name "pink-eye"). Secondary bacterial infections occur leading to various complications, including pneumonia.

Treatment

The treatment of these viral respiratory diseases is unsatisfactory, as with many other diseases associated with viral infections. Animals should be kept warm and well nursed, rugged if necessary and legs bandaged. Fresh drinking water should be readily available. Antibiotics and sulphonamides are used to control secondary bacterial infections.

INFECTIOUS EQUINE BRONCHITIS

THIS is an infectious bronchitis commonly seen in racing stables, hence the common name "Newmarket Cough". It is also known as contagious equine catarrh and infectious equine cough. The disease occurs in most countries of the world, including Australia and New Zealand. Although not a serious disease, it causes interruption in training and, if an affected horse is not rested and given nursing attention, may lead to a more serious form of bronchitis and bronchopneumonia.

Cause

The disease is believed to be caused by a virus and is very contagious. It spreads rapidly, apparently by inhalation, in racing stables or where a number of horses are closely confined. Secondary bacterial infection, although not common, can complicate the disease. The incubation period is short, usually about three days.

Symptoms

There is at first a mild temperature (103° F.), slight depression, some loss of appetite, watery discharge from the nose, and soreness of the lymph glands of the throat on palpation. There is no reddening of, nor discharge from, the eyes. These symptoms pass off after three or four days by which time, however, a persistent hacking cough has developed, which may last for several weeks. There are frequent paroxysms of hard dry coughing.

Treatment

Good nursing and rest are usually all that is required in the treatment of this mild but distressing disease. An electuary on the tongue, such as that recommended under *Bronchitis*, is helpful in relieving the coughing. The feed should be dampened to avoid dustiness. Care should be taken that the animal is only worked lightly during convalescence. Affected horses should be isolated to prevent spread of the disease. Should complications occur, no time should be lost in obtaining professional assistance so that antibiotic treatment may be carried out.

JAUNDICE (Icterus)

JAUNDICE, icterus or "yellows" is not a specific disease but is a clinical symptom which arises from disorders of the liver and biliary system and also in association with other diseases. There is a yellowish discoloration of the visible mucous membranes such as the eyes, nose, mouth and genital organs. In white or light-coloured horses even the skin may show this yellow tint. The urine is bright yellow or even greenish in colour, the dung is a dirty-grey colour and constipation is usually present. Although jaundice occurs as a common symptom of certain well-known diseases, it can occur as a symptom of almost any inflammatory disease accompanied by high fever. Obstructive jaundice, due to occlusion of the bile duct by calculi or from other causes—the horse has no gall bladder—is not common in the horse, but can occur. *Neonatal jaundice* is sometimes seen in foals. The treatment for jaundice depends entirely on the cause.

JOINT-ILL (Navel-ill)

JOINT-ILL (navel-ill or polyarthritis) is a serious disease of foals and, prior to the advent of antibiotic drugs, was responsible for many deaths. It arises from infection through the navel shortly after birth, and sometimes whilst the foal is still in the uterus. The infection spreads to various organs of the body causing a variety of disease conditions, and occasionally a fatal septicaemia. It commonly attacks various joints leading to the term *joint-ill*.

Cause

A large number of organisms have been found to be associated with the development of this disease complex. It is well recognized that the disease is more prone to occur when the mare foals in a "foaling-box" or stable, or when assistance is given to the mare when foaling. It is far less likely to occur when the mare foals in a wellgrassed paddock and without human interference.

Symptoms

In most cases symptoms appear within the first few weeks of life, depending on the mode and type of infection. If infection has

109

occurred in the uterus, the foal may be born dead or in a weakened condition, is fevered, obviously sick and disinclined to suck its mother. Death commonly occurs in two or three days. When infection occurs shortly after birth, symptoms are generally shown in seven to eight days, sometimes longer, depending on the type of infection. There may be little or no evidence of infection at the navel with certain types of organisms. On the other hand, when the infection is due to pus-forming organisms, there is abscess formation at the navel. The foal is depressed and listless, has a temperature above normal and shows increased respiration and pulse rates. Swelling of the joints with accompanying lameness occurs, particularly of the stifle and hock, but also of other joints such as the knee, shoulder, elbow and fetlock. The joint swelling becomes hot, tense and painful and after a few days may burst and discharge a serous, blood-stained fluid and sometimes pus. Alternatively, the swelling may regress, the heat subside and the joint appear normal again, but such a joint may cause lameness later in life. In addition to fatal septicaemia, the disease is particularly serious when abscess formation occurs in the lungs, liver and other internal organs.

Treatment

This disease in foals is far too serious for any attempt at treatment by the horse-owner. Immediately any symptoms are shown which suggest navel infection, the services of a veterinary surgeon should be obtained in order that antibiotic, sulphonamide and perhaps cortisone treatment can be commenced without delay. Any other forms of treatment are unlikely to give satisfactory results.

Prevention

It will be obvious that prevention lies mainly in good hygiene at foaling time. The best environment is that of a well-grassed, spelled paddock. In Australia, most mares do foal in the paddock and when they do so and the navel cord breaks naturally and no assistance is necessary at foaling, joint-ill is unlikely to occur. It is very important that the young foal should receive the colostrum in the first milk from the mother, as this contains antibodies which protect the foal against infection by various organisms. Should the foal be weak at birth, it should be assisted to the mare's teats and encouraged to suck, but the navel should not be interfered with. If it is necessary to render assistance at foaling, the strictest hygiene should be maintained. The fingernails of the attendant should be cut short and the hands and arms washed thoroughly in hot water and soap to which some antiseptic has been added. The external genitals and tail of the mare should be washed in antiseptic solution and other precautionary measures taken to prevent infection, particularly if the cord is broken

110

in the course of the manipulations or has to be cut with sterile scissors. The application of strong antiseptics to the navel stump is likely to do more harm than good, as this retards healing and may encourage bacterial infection. Dusting the stump with sulphanilamide dusting powder would be preferable to the use of tincture of iodine as formerly recommended. The umbilical cord should be handled as little as possible.

KNEES, BROKEN

"BROKEN KNEES" is the term applied to any wound inflicted on a horse's knees by falling or otherwise lacerating the area. It is referred to specifically not only because of its common occurrence, but because scars or blemishes on the knees affect the value of the horse. The so-called horse's knee is not actually the knee at all. It corresponds to the human wrist and is composed of two rows of bones, three in each row and a seventh one placed at the back of the upper row of bones.

Causes

Bad conformation may be responsible for a horse stumbling and injuring the knees; illness, weariness, careless driving, riding, and handling of the horse are other causes. A blemished knee is always looked upon with suspicion, even though it may be claimed that it was caused purely by accident.

Symptoms

These vary from mere abrasions of the skin to damage of tendons and oil sheaths with infection. This may result in varying degrees of lameness, which may not appear until exercise.

Treatment

Clean the wound by irrigating thoroughly with some mild, non-irritating antiseptic solution, such as *Dettol* or *Cetavlon* or normal saline solution (1 oz. salt to a pint of boiled water). Allow to dry and cover with some soothing antiseptic ointment, apply oiled gauze and bandage lightly. Some excellent ointments incorporating modern drugs and vitamin A are available. Sulphanilamide powder is commonly used to dust the wound. If the injury is not severe it is preferable, after cleaning the wound, simply to dust it with this powder and not to bandage. Repeated bathing of the wound once it has been cleaned is undesirable. The objective in treatment is to get the wound to heal as quickly as possible with a minimum amount of scar tissue. A cradle may have to be placed on the horse to prevent him biting the knee when it is healing. When the joint capsule has been pene-

111

trated, professional assistance should be sought. In any case, irrespective of the extent of the injury, a tetanus antitoxin injection is desirable. Treatment under veterinary supervision will minimize the possibility of a large scar.

KIDNEYS—INFLAMMATION OF (Nephritis)

CONTRARY to the general opinion of horsemen, it is comparatively rare for the horse's kidneys to be primarily diseased. Except in old horses, acute and chronic inflammations of the kidneys do not commonly occur.

See *Colic*

Causes

Diseases of other organs of the body such as the liver, lungs and heart, may lead to kidney inflammation. Among the predisposing causes of acute nephritis are over-exertion, falls, blows, and prolonged exposure to cold and draughts which lower the resistance of the kidneys to bacterial infection.

The administration of certain diuretic drugs for supposed kidney complaints, and the use of turpentine and resins in drenches may cause inflammation of the kidneys. Heavy blistering with liquid blisters containing cantharides is sometimes responsible for the condition. Chronic nephritis may follow an acute condition and is also seen as a complication of certain specific infectious diseases, and in old age.

Symptoms

Alteration in the quality and quantity of the urine—usually a small quantity at a time, of a high colour and sometimes mixed with pus and blood; arching of the back; continued straining; stiff and straddling gait; pain over the loins on slight pressure; swelling of the legs and weakness. In chronic cases, there is poor or irregular appetite; loss of condition; flabbiness of the muscles; paleness of the mucous membranes of the eyes and nose and, in severe cases, skin eruptions. Following diminution in the amount of urine passed, indicating disease of both kidneys, death follows from uraemia.

Treatment

The treatment of diseases of the urinary system is essentially a matter for a veterinarian, and involves the use of urinary antiseptics, antibiotics and sedatives. An acute case of nephritis might be given home treatment by administering a saline purgative drench (*Epsom* or *Glauber's* salts—8 to 10 oz. in 1 pint of water). A quart of liquid

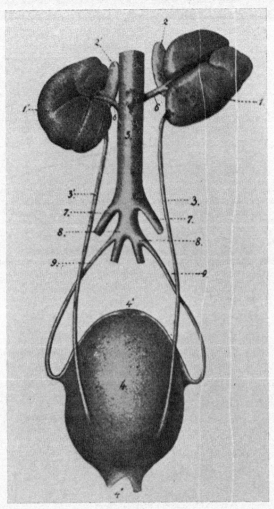

Fig. 51 Urinary Organs of the Horse.
(After Leiserings Atlas in Sisson-Grossman, Anatomy of the Domestic Animals, 4th edition. Philadelphia, W. B. Saunders Co., 1953)

paraffin may be given instead of the salts. Blankets saturated with hot water should be applied over the loins and the horse rested and kept warm by rugging. If the horse shows signs of much pain, $\frac{3}{4}$ oz. of chlorodyne may be given in water two or three times a day but discontinued as soon as the pain is relieved. Turpentine and nitrate (nitre) should *not* be given.

113

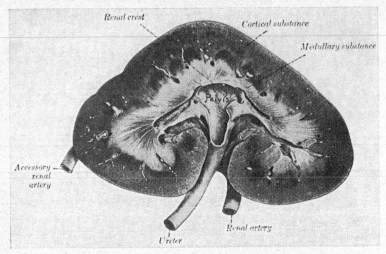

Fig. 52　Frontal (Horizontal) Section of Kidney of the Horse.
(From Sisson-Grossman: Anatomy of the Domestic Animals, 4th edition. Philadelphia. W. B. Saunders Co., 1953)

The horse may be given linseed tea to drink, and the diet should consist mainly of bran mashes and green feed. Care is necessary during convalescence to see that the animal is kept warm and not subjected to active exertion for some time after all symptoms have subsided.

KIMBERLEY OR WALKABOUT DISEASE

A FATAL disease of horses occurs in the Kimberley Division of Western Australia and in the Northern Territory of Australia. It has been the subject of considerable research.

Cause

A native plant *Crotalaria retusa*, which grows in the low-lying areas of the main river systems which are subject to flooding, has been found to be the poison plant which causes the disease.

Symptoms

It is called Walkabout Disease because the affected animals walk in a straight line into fences and other obstructions and may stand for hours pushing at the obstacle. They also walk into creeks and rivers and stumble over logs. The earlier symptoms are those of sleepiness, irritability, depraved appetite and yawning. Affected animals also show incoordination of movement, and twitching of head and neck muscles. They are reluctant to lie down, and when

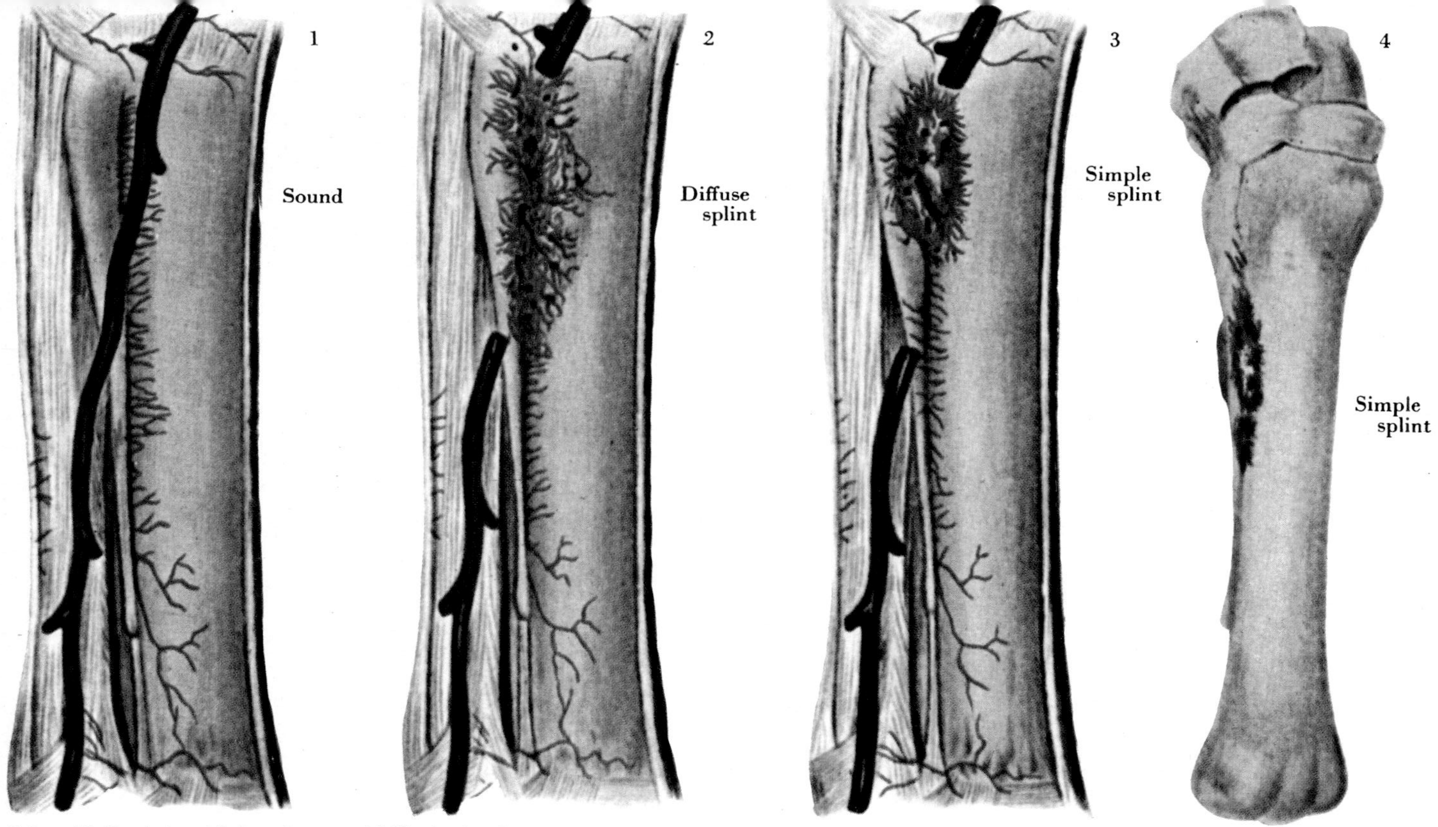

Haines, del. Nos. 1, 2, and 3, from Auzoux model, No. 4, original.

PLATE 1. SPLINT (*United States Department of Agriculture*)

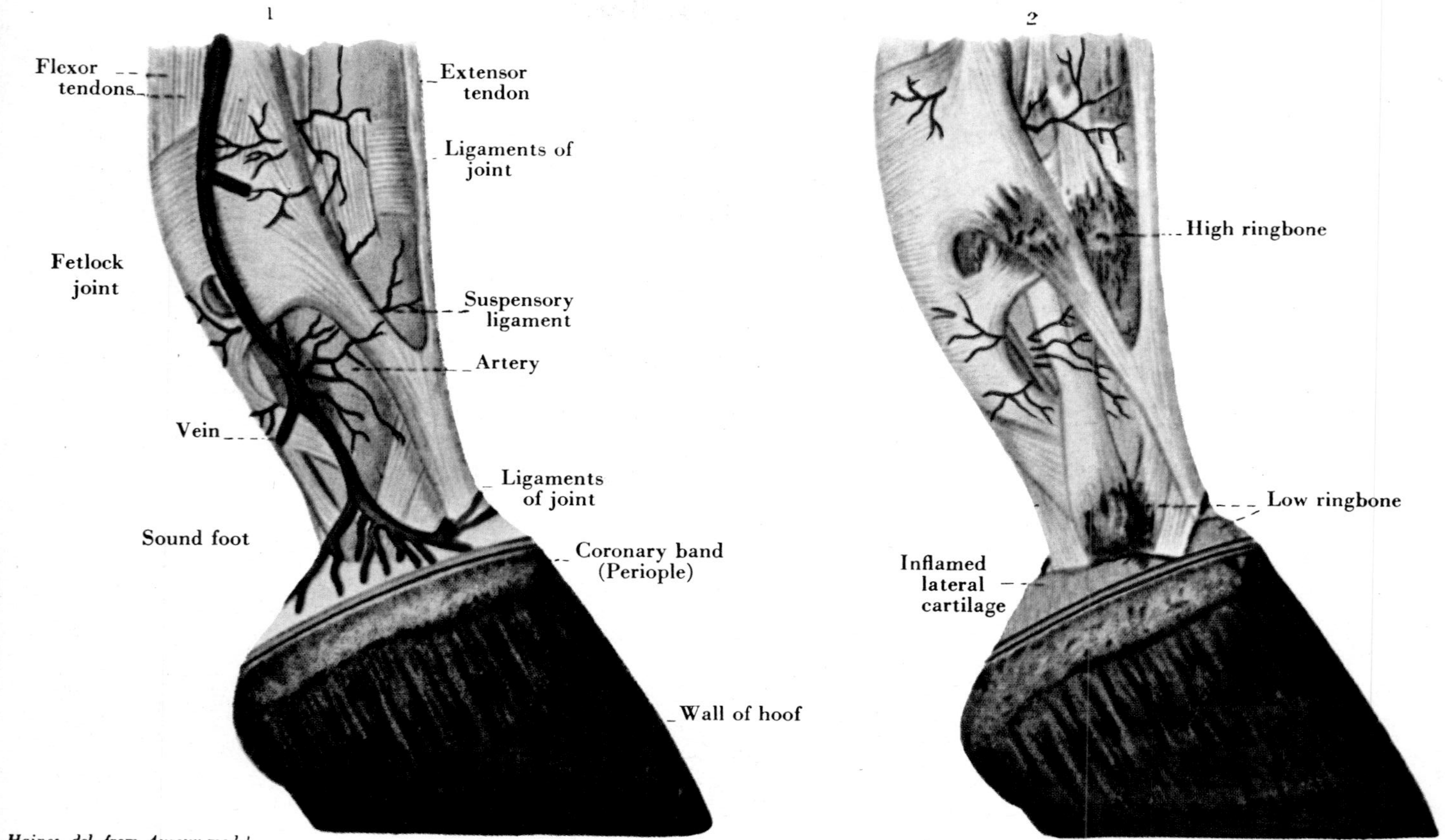
1
2
Flexor tendons
Extensor tendon
Ligaments of joint
Fetlock joint
Suspensory ligament
Artery
Vein
Ligaments of joint
Sound foot
Coronary band (Periople)
Wall of hoof
High ringbone
Low ringbone
Inflamed lateral cartilage

Haines, del. from Auzoux model.

PLATE 2. (Left) SOUND FOOT, (right) RING BONE (*United States Department of Agriculture*)

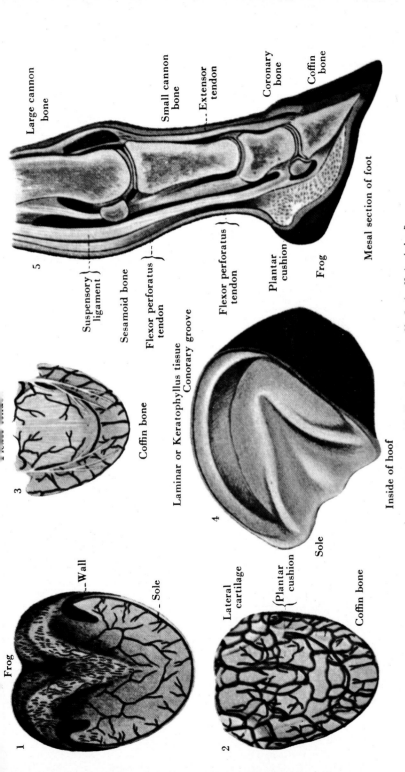

Frog

Wall

Sole

1

Lateral
cartilage

Plantar
cushion

Coffin bone

2

Coffin bone

3

Laminar or Keratophyllus tissue
Conorary groove

Inside of hoof

Sole

4

Large cannon
bone

Small cannon
bone

Extensor
tendon

Coronary
bone

Coffin
bone

Suspensory
ligament

Sesamoid bone

Flexor perforatus
tendon

Flexor perforatus
tendon

Plantar
cushion

Frog

Mesal section of foot

5

Haines, del. Nos. 1, 2, and 3, from model. No. 4, from nature. No. 5, after Hering (colored).

PLATE 3. ANATOMY OF FOOT (*United States Department of Agriculture*)

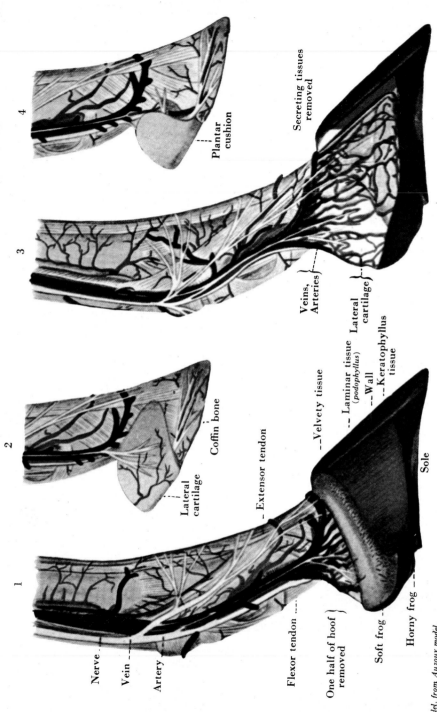

1

Nerve
Vein
Artery

Flexor tendon
One half of hoof } removed
Soft frog
Horny frog

Sole

2

Lateral cartilage

Coffin bone

Extensor tendon

Velvety tissue

Laminar tissue (podophyllus)
Wall
Keratophyllus tissue

3

Veins, Arteries }
Lateral cartilage }

4

Plantar cushion

Secreting tissues removed

Haines, del. from Auzoux model.

down may be unable to rise without assistance. The urine is coffee-coloured or red and symptoms of jaundice may be shown.

The "walkabout" symptoms extend over a period of weeks or months with progressive and extreme emaciation. Eventually the horse goes down, is unable to rise, goes into a coma and death occurs. The main post-mortem finding is cirrhosis of the liver.

Treatment

There is no known treatment.

Prevention

The only preventive measure that can be adopted is to endeavour to prevent horses grazing over areas which are subject to flooding and where the plant grows.

Differential Diagnosis

Kimberley horse disease must be differentiated from another horse disease known as *Birdsville Disease*, which occurs also in the Northern Territory of Australia and in western Queensland and the north of South Australia. This disease is caused by a poison plant *Indigofera enneaphylla* and the symptoms are in some respects similar to Kimberley horse disease. Early symptoms are sleepiness and incoordination of gait in which the front feet are lifted high from the ground and there is some absence of control of the hind limbs. Horses affected with Birdsville disease are inclined to stand still rather than to wander, and if forced to move are inclined to drag the hind limbs. Chronically affected cases drag the hind limbs constantly and wear away the horn of the feet. Mildly affected cases may recover, but usually an affected horse, which does not die from starvation or thirst, is left with some chronic disability. There is no effective treatment and all that can be done is to deny horses access to the Indigofera plant, if possible.

LAMENESS

Books have been written on lameness and its diagnosis in the horse. Lameness may be defined as any irregularity or derangement of the function of locomotion, irrespective of its cause. Detection of the cause of the lameness is often very difficult, even for a veterinarian, who has the advantage of a knowledge of the anatomy of the horse. It is easy enough to detect the cause of lameness when some obvious injury, such as a wound or open joint, exists, but quite another matter when a horse just "goes lame". Slight lameness is more difficult to diagnose than more pronounced lameness. In horses, most causes of lameness occur at or below the knee and hock, whereas

I

lameness in the shoulder and hip are comparatively rare. Where no apparent and sufficient cause of trouble can be detected and the affected limb has been recognized, the foot must be thoroughly examined and, if necessary, the shoe removed to further the examination.

Detection of the Seat of Lameness

Close observation of a horse at rest or as he stands in a stable will often reveal the affected leg. If he "points" one fore limb, the trouble will probably be in this leg. If the trouble is in both fore feet, the horse is inclined to "point" each leg alternately. Watching a horse turn in a stable may show that he drops on one side, thus indicating lameness on the other side, either in front or behind.

Usually the best method of detecting the seat of lameness is to have the animal led away by a halter and then trotted slowly on hard ground. The horse should be observed from various points—in front, from behind and from each side. When an animal is lame, it takes as much weight as possible off the injured or painful limb and places it on the opposite one. The extra weight placed on the sound limb causes irregularity of action. In the case of foreleg lameness, it will be noted that when the horse is trotted towards the observer, the animal nods its head when the foot of the sound limb strikes the ground and the head rises when the foot of the lame leg is on the ground. If no abnormality of action is seen in the forelegs, the action of the hind legs should be observed as the horse is trotted away. In hind-leg lameness, the hock of the sound leg rises higher and dips lower than that of the lame one, and the hip drops on the sound side.

Briefly then, when the horse nods its head as the foot of the right foreleg strikes the ground, the animal is lame in the left foreleg, and if it dips the hock and drops the hip as the foot of the right hind leg strikes the ground, it is lame in the left hind leg. If the nodding of the head and drooping of the hip are on the near or left side, the lameness is on the off or right side. When the animal is lame in both forelegs, it takes short strides and walks in a rather stilted fashion with what is commonly referred to as a "proppy" gait. Double hind-limb lameness may also be indicated by short strides and stiffness of movement suggestive of injury to the loins. Backing is difficult in these cases.

A horse which is very lame in one foreleg may appear to be lame in the diagonal hind leg also when trotting away. This can be very deceptive to the inexperienced observer.

When there is a combination of fore- and hind-limb lameness, the detection of the seat of lameness becomes much more difficult and usually requires the assistance of a veterinarian, both for detection and diagnosis of the cause of the lameness.

When a horse has been found to be lame in a given leg, it becomes necessary to decide what structure is involved and this is not always easy. It may be possible to localize the seat of the trouble by noting the way in which the lame leg is performing its functions; by observing the motions of the whole leg, especially of the various joints; by minutely examining every part of the leg; by observing the outlines and by feeling for heat and testing for sensitiveness. All these will be a guide to a correct localization of the trouble, but a hasty conclusion should not be formed, and it must never be forgotten that all parts of the foot must be carefully examined. It is not at all uncommon for lameness to have an apparent location elsewhere when the foot is the true seat of the trouble.

The various disease conditions which cause lameness are dealt with alphabetically throughout the book.

LAMINITIS
See *Founder*

LAMPAS (Palatitis)
LAMPAS is a congestion and swelling of the mucous membrane of the hard palate just behind the upper incisor teeth and to which, in the past, undue attention has been paid by horsemen. Lampas is not a disease entity and does not affect the health of the horse. Some congestion of the spongy tissue of the hard palate always occurs when the horse is feeding. When, however, there is some irritation in the mouth, such as in stomatitis, or there is congestion associated with shedding of the temporary teeth and eruption of the permanent incisor teeth, the prominence of the hard palate may persist temporarily owing to the increased blood supply to the part. It is this condition which is commonly referred to as lampas in young horses. The condition is sometimes seen in old horses when again it is usually associated with dentition but also with digestive disturbance.

Examination of the mouth shows the front bars of the hard palate extending below the level of the incisor teeth, causing the horse to feed badly while the swelling persists.

Treatment
Under no circumstances should the swelling of the palate be interfered with in any way by lancing, scarification or the barbarous practice of cauterizing the area. The horse might be given a mild

117

purgative drench to advantage and be fed a few bran mashes. Some loose hay should be fed to provide massage to the part, otherwise soft food should be given. The swelling usually subsides without further medicinal treatment. As a local application, a simple astringent lotion such as ½ oz. of potassium chlorate, borax or alum in a pint of water may be dabbed on the palate three or four times a day. Dental irregularities in old horses should be corrected and attention directed to the diet.

LARYNGITIS

LARYNGITIS or inflammation of the larynx is usually associated with some general infection of the upper respiratory tract, including tracheitis, rhinitis and sometimes bronchitis, or with certain infectious diseases such as strangles. Simple or acute catarrhal laryngitis commonly follows some predisposing factor, such as exposure to cold or dampness, inhalation of dust, smoke, gases, the lodging of foreign bodies such as grass seeds in the larynx, and careless use of the stomach tube. These factors bring about a catarrhal inflammation of the mucous membrane of the larynx, accompanied not infrequently by considerable oedematous swelling. Inflammation of the larynx is commonly complicated by pharyngitis or inflammation of the pharynx, constituting what is popularly known as "sore throat".

Symptoms

These depend on the severity of the inflammation of the mucous membranes of the area. The outstanding symptom is a frequent, short, dry and harsh cough, which later becomes more prolonged and is accompanied by a discharge from both nostrils.

Pressure over the laryngeal region with the fingers causes pain and attacks of coughing. The respiration is normal while the animal is at rest and the laryngitis remains localized. Not infrequently, however, it is complicated by bronchitis when there is an alteration in the normal respiratory rate. Fever is generally absent or slight, but the appetite is somewhat diminished. The horse may have difficulty in swallowing, and water and sometimes food is returned through the nostrils. There may be some swelling in the throat region and the head may be "poked out". Redness of the mucous membrane of the nose is commonly seen and there may be a harsh rasping snore. Diagnosis is based on the cough and the sensitiveness of the throat region. The prognosis is favourable in cases of simple laryngitis, the course of the disease being about ten days, sometimes longer. The after effects of a severe attack of laryngitis are a chronic cough, whistling and roaring.

Treatment

Simple laryngitis frequently responds to home treatment. The animal should be kept warm, but if stabled the ventilation should be adequate without draughts. If the weather is cold, Newmarket bandages might be applied to the legs for warmth and support. The horse should be given soft feed, such as bran mashes, scalded oats, linseed gruel and the like. Dry feed should be dampened to control dust. Steam inhalations by holding the horse's head over a bucket of hot water containing 2 tablespoons of *Friar's* balsam afford relief to the animal. Drenching should be avoided. External treatment is of little value, although hot packs to the throat region followed by camphorated oil or camphor and soap liniment, gently rubbed into the throat, may be of assistance in reducing inflammation. Electuaries of various types, to soothe the inflamed mucous membranes, may be placed on the tongue or molar teeth with a flat smooth stick every three or four hours. The following is a useful electuary: Extract belladonna 1 oz., chlorate of potash 2 oz., boracic acid 1 oz., glycerine 2 oz., honey to make 8 oz. Dose: 1 to 2 tablespoons. Finally, antibiotics and sulphonamides may be used under veterinary supervision if the case does not respond to the simple treatments, or should complications occur.

LEG MANGE ("Itchy Heel")

LEG mange is a fairly common parasitic disease of the skin and in the days when draught horses were used on farms, was the cause of much damage to fences as a result of horses rubbing their heels on the wires. Although the condition is mainly confined to the legs below the hocks and knees, it occasionally reaches to the inner thighs and armpits. It may appear along the belly, and the muzzle and nose may be affected as a result of the horse biting at the legs.

Cause

The disease is caused by a minute mange mite, *Chorioptes equi*, which is picked up by close contact with infested horses or from fences, posts, stumps and so on, recently contaminated by them. It is usual, therefore, for several horses on a farm or riding school to be affected in varying degree.

Under warm conditions eggs laid by the female hatch in about three days and burrow under the surface layer of the skin, feeding on skin scales and other debris. The young mites reach sexual maturity in about six days and begin to breed, so that the mite population increases rapidly in spite of the fact that the average life of the mite is only about fourteen days. Since warmth favours the

119

rapid multiplication of these parasites, the condition is more apparent during the summer months, becoming dormant during a cold dry winter, only to flare up again the following summer.

As already pointed out, infestation by the parasite of leg mange is mainly confined to the lower extremities of the legs and especially the hind legs. In this way it differs from other mange parasites of horses, not known to be present in Australia, which spread all over the body or affect the mane and tail.

Symptoms

The activities of the mites cause a reddening of the skin around the affected areas from which moisture oozes to form hard crusts. Later the skin becomes thickened and thrown into ridges. Intense irritation occurs, which is shown by the affected horse stamping, pawing, kicking and rubbing the pastern with the opposite foot or biting at the affected area. The horse is inclined to back up against fences, stumps and logs and rub its heels or backs of the legs against these objects. This constant rubbing causes the hair on the legs to be worn and ragged in appearance. If the condition is not treated, serious complications may result, such as greasy heel or damage to the foot from stamping, and even fractures may occur.

Diagnosis of the disease may be confirmed by microscopic examination of skin scrapings from the affected areas for the presence of mange mites.

Treatment

Clip the affected areas closely and wash with warm lime-sulphur (containing 1 per cent polysulphide). Lime-sulphur concentrates are prepared by a number of firms as orchard sprays and are guaranteed to contain 20 per cent polysulphide. If this concentrate is diluted 1 in 20, it makes a satisfactory wash. If large numbers of horses have to be treated, this 1 per cent solution can be used in a foot-bath. Re-treatment should be given in one week to 10 days and still further treatments may be necessary at the same intervals to clear up the condition. Older treatments, such as 1 part sulphur to 4 parts lard, applied warm, are not as effective as the warm lime-sulphur wash.

Stables and other premises should be disinfected and attention given to rugs, brushes and harness which may remain infective for up to three weeks.

LICE

HORSES are commonly infested by two species of lice, the horse sucking louse (*Haematopinus asini*) and the horse biting louse

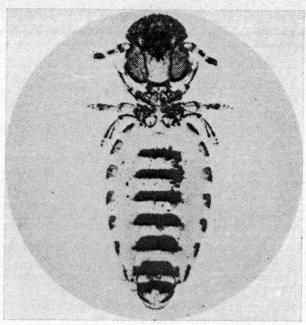

Fig. 53   A biting louse of the horse, *Damalinia equi*.
(From Insects Affecting Livestock. F. H. S. Roberts)

(*Damalinia equi*). These lice have similar life histories, the eggs hatching in 8 to 10 days or a little longer. The louse spends the whole of its life upon the host, which it does not leave unless to transfer to another horse, and which it can readily do when there is close contact between horses, or it is forcibly removed or reaches the ground with fallen hair. The sucking louse may remain alive off the host for 2 to 3 days and the biting louse for as long as 10 days. Eggs attached to fallen hair remain viable for 20 days away from the host, hatch under favourable conditions and the young lice survive for a further 2 to 3 days. Harness, saddles, rugs and grooming utensils may harbour the lice and eggs for similar periods. The parasites increase rapidly during the winter when the hair is long and decrease when the hair is shed in the spring. Sucking lice are more commonly found at the base of the mane and tail, while biting lice favour the lower parts of the body and jaws, but also congregate on the back and flanks. In heavy infestations lice extend all over the body.

Symptoms

The irritation caused by lice causes the horse to stamp, kick and rub against objects. The hair is rubbed off in patches and the skin

121

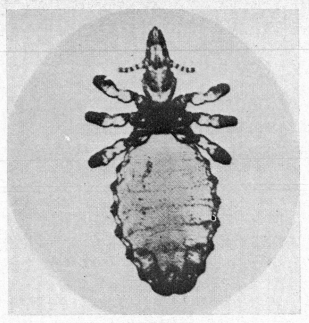

Fig. 54 The Sucking louse of the horse, *Haematopinus asini*.
(From Insects Affecting Livestock. F. H. S. Roberts)

may be bruised and lacerated. Heavy infestation with sucking lice causes blood loss and weakens the animal, and is often one of the reasons for poor condition or "poverty".

Treatment

Horses with heavy coats should be clipped and the clippings burnt. Dipping or spraying are the usual methods of applying insecticides for the control of lice infestation and, in the case of horses, owing to the lack of dipping facilities, spraying is mainly carried out. This must be done thoroughly, taking care that the horse is wetted all over. Because insecticides cannot be relied upon to kill 'he eggs or nits, or to remain toxic long enough to kill all the young lice which hatch from the eggs, it is necessary to repeat the spraying in 14 days. Various insecticides are used in dips or sprays but the organic phosphorus compounds such as *diazinon, Asuntol, Nankor* and *Ethion* now recommended for the control of cattle lice, are to be preferred. The manufacturer's instructions should be carefully followed. Various insecticide dusts are used where it is undesirable to wet the horse during cold weather, but, as better results are obtained

122

with thorough spraying, it is desirable to spray in the autumn so that the horse enters the winter free from infestation.

The stable or shed in which the horse is accommodated should be thoroughly cleaned down and bedding and sweepings burned. The woodwork and floor should then be well sprayed with an effective insecticide, paying particular attention to spaces between boards. Care should be taken that excess of spray is not left in depressions, and that the premises have thoroughly dried before being re-occupied. Treatment of harness, rugs, brushes and other contaminated articles should not be overlooked.

LYMPHANGITIS (SPORADIC) ("Bigleg", "Weed", "Monday Morning Disease")

LYMPHANGITIS means inflammation and enlargement of the lymph gland. Although there are other diseases of the lymphatic system, such as ulcerative lymphangitis, epizootic lymphangitis, and glanders, a specific non-contagious disease of horses known as sporadic lymphangitis has been recognized for a long time and is mentioned in the oldest veterinary books. Although in the past the disease was more commonly seen in heavy draught horses, it can occur in all types of horses.

The disease must be differentiated from azoturia (*paralytic myoglobinuria*).

Cause

The actual cause of this disease is not known, although the circumstances under which it occurs are fairly well understood. Some investigators consider that the disease develops as a result of infection by certain common organisms, and a disturbance in the protein balance has been considered a predisposing cause. Sporadic lymphangitis occurs more commonly in horses receiving full rations rich in protein and doing little or no work. It commonly occurs when horses have been spelled over the week-end and full working rations supplied, hence the common name "Monday morning disease". The condition appears to be due to partial stasis of the circulation and lymph flow of the leg, which in some cases could be due to infection of superficial wounds and ulcers on the lower parts of the limbs. There would appear to be little doubt that lack of exercise combined with a high protein diet are important predisposing causes.

Symptoms

The disease commences suddenly and is accompanied by high fever (105° to 106° F.), shivering, rapid pulse rate and respiration, followed by swelling of one or both hind legs. The animal stands in a dejected manner, not eating and is constipated. Usually only one hind leg is affected, the limb being swollen and hot and distended lymph-vessels can be felt as cords running up the inside of the leg. In the early stages of the disease, pain is shown when these vessels are pressed. The swelling spreads from above downwards, gradually surrounding the whole leg until it reaches the foot. It is often sharply defined from healthy structures above. Lameness is very pronounced and the horse shows evidence of pain when made to walk. Swelling may sometimes occur in the front legs. The acute stage of the disease generally lasts about 3 days; the fever abates; the swelling recedes and becomes less painful. Occasionally abscesses develop in the lymph glands and vessels. Complete recovery takes about two weeks, but if the swelling does not receive prompt attention, it may persist long enough for a permanent fibrotic enlargement to be produced in the leg. Even with the best of attention, some permanent increase in the size of the leg generally remains after a severe attack of the disease. A horse which has once been affected with the disease is liable to recurrent attacks.

Treatment

Professional assistance should be obtained in order that injections of appropriate antibiotics can be given in the early stages of the disease to control the infection. Local treatment of the swollen leg or legs by fomenting frequently with hot water is very important and contributes considerably to the animal's recovery. Gentle upward massage of the limb should be given. This may be followed by the application of cold water or the free use of an astringent lotion such as "white lotion" (1 oz. zinc sulphate and 1 oz. lead acetate in a pint of water) after first drying the limb. It is advisable to bandage the leg or legs fairly tightly in the intervals between fomentations and massage. The horse should be given a laxative drench, such as 2 pints of liquid paraffin or a pint of raw linseed oil, and 1 to 3 drachms of potassium nitrate (nitre) twice a day in the drinking water (using a bucket), or in bran mashes. As soon as the horse can bear weight on the leg, a few minutes' exercise several times a day is desirable. The feed should consist of freshly prepared bran mashes, greenstuff and a small amount of good hay while the horse is sick. It is necessary that an adequate supply of drinking water be readily available as the horse is usually very thirsty. The return to normal hard feed should be very gradual. Complete rest for at least a fortnight is usually necessary in uncomplicated cases and the horse should not be returned to work until all lameness has disappeared.

Prevention lies in cutting down the feed supply of spelling horses, especially concentrates, which can well be dispensed with when the horse is not working, and by substituting instead a ration of lucerne hay. Horses brought in from grass for hand-feeding should be introduced to concentrates gradually.

MANGE

OTHER than leg mange caused by the mange mite *Chorioptes equi*, the only other type of mange which affects horses in Australia is that known as otacariasis or ear mange, caused by the mange mite *Psoroptes hippotis*. It has been recorded in Queensland and New South Wales but is not yet of economic importance. Treatment with BHC is said to be effective.

Sarcoptic mange or scabies in horses, which is prevalent in overseas countries, does not occur in Australia.

See *Leg Mange*

MASTITIS (Inflammation of the Udder)

MASTITIS means inflammation of the mammary gland, regardless of the cause. This condition is comparatively rare in the mare, although sometimes the udder becomes painfully distended prior to or after foaling and a doughy swelling, pitting on pressure, extends forward along the abdomen. This may recede or a more serious condition develops, when one or both glands become enlarged, hot, tense and painful and the milk dries up or is replaced by a watery or reddish fluid. The mare walks lamely, goes off her feed, has a temperature and shows all symptoms of a general constitutional disturbance.

Cause

The latter condition is of bacterial origin and its severity depends on the type of infection. Sometimes the infection leads to gangrene of the udder or results in death from septicaemia.

Treatment

In the early stages, hot fomentations and active massage with a little olive oil in the palm of the hand, and frequent drawing off of milk by hand may bring about rapid improvement. If this fails, professional attention should be obtained immediately, as infection is likely. When the disease persists, milk samples should be submitted to a veterinary laboratory, preferably by a veterinarian, for determination of the type of infection. Subsequent treatment with antibiotics will depend largely on the laboratory report. If an antibiotic cream is to be injected into the udder, it should be noted that the mare has three separate ducts opening on the summit of each teat and each has to be carefully injected.

MELANOMA

A MELANOMA is a malignant neoplasm or tumour which contains melanin, a black or dark brown pigment. These occur more frequently in old grey horses, although they do occur in horses of other colours, especially in horses after 10 years of age when the coat begins to turn white. The condition is associated with abnormal pigmentary deposits. The tumours commonly occur under the root of the tail and sometimes on the upper surface, and about the anus, sheath and crest. From these situations, they spread to neighbouring lymphatic glands and then, by metastasis, to the spleen, lungs and other internal organs.

Treatment

This is unsatisfactory even by operation and it is better to destroy the animal.

METRITIS (Inflammation of the Uterus)

THE TERM used to describe inflammation of the uterus (womb) is metritis. In the mare, acute metritis most commonly occurs after foaling, but occasionally it occurs in late pregnancy when it usually results in the death of the foetus and sometimes also of the mare.

Cause

Inflammations of the uterus are the result of bacterial infections, which usually occur at normal or assisted foaling, more particularly the latter, but can also occur by the extension of infections from other parts of the genital tract. Unless great cleanliness is observed when rendering assistance to a mare at foaling time, infection can be carried into the uterus by the hands or arms of the operator or by the ropes, instruments or other apparatus used to assist birth of the foal. Further, if the mare fails to "clean" properly and a portion of the "afterbirth" is retained in the uterus, this soon putrefies, leading to infection and inflammation of the uterus.

Symptoms

Acute inflammation of the uterus usually results in systemic as well as local symptoms. In the mare, this disease is a serious condition and is often fatal. Within 24 to 72 hours after foaling, the mare exhibits uneasiness; fever; shivering; accelerated breathing; arched back; stiff movements of body and looks back at the flanks. A discharge occurs from the vulva, which may at first be watery, reddish or yellow, but later becomes thicker and more abundant and may be foetid. The mare goes off her feed, loses interest in the foal and may lose her milk. She maintains a standing position. Stiffness of move-

126

ment and difficulty of lifting the feet from the ground indicate that inflammation of the sensitive laminae of the foot (founder) has occurred, this being commonly associated with acute metritis. Other complications, such as inflammation of the udder, bladder, vagina and, still more serious, peritonitis and pneumonia are likely to occur.

If the mare survives, chronic metritis may supervene upon the acute attack and be the reason why a mare does not subsequently get in foal.

Treatment

The treatment of an acute case of metritis is essentially a matter for a veterinarian. Satisfactory treatment cannot usually be carried out by the horse-owner and usually more harm than good is done in attempting to douche out the uterus, frequently with inadequate instruments and lack of knowledge of the anatomy of the parts. Flushing out the vagina is a simple matter and will remove discharges that have passed through the cervical canal (neck of the uterus), but the fluid does not get into the uterus, the seat of the infection. Further, if fluid is injected into the uterus, it must be siphoned out afterwards. A veterinarian, in addition to inserting suitable antibiotic pessaries into the uterus—a superior method of treatment to the use of antiseptic fluids—will also give large doses of antibiotics sub·cutaneously and intramuscularly, and possibly also sulphonamide drugs by the mouth. In addition, stilboestrol may be administered to stimulate activity of the uterus in the case of retained membranes.

The mare should be well nursed, given laxative food, such as bran mashes and green feed, and should be rugged if the weather is cold, when complications such as founder and pneumonia can occur.

See *Founder* and *Pneumonia*

MYOSITIS—ACUTE ("Tying-up" or "Cording-up")

THE TERMS "tying-up" and "cording-up" are commonly used in racing stables to describe a muscular disorder, the cause of which is not thoroughly understood. The condition is similar to paralytic myoglobinuria, commonly known as "Monday morning sickness" which was once frequently seen in working draught horses. (See *Azoturia.*) It is sometimes called *atypical myoglobinuria*. The disease is seen more particularly in race horses and light horses under heavy exercise or training. It can also occur in the heavier breeds of horses. Whereas paralytic myoglobinuria (Azoturia) commonly occurs when the horse is put to work following a short period of idleness whilst being maintained on full working rations, "tying-up" or "cording-up" occurs following strenuous exercise, or after a hard day's work, in horses that are in training and being fed rations consistent with the work performed.

Symptoms

The term myositis means inflammation of a muscle and this is essentially what happens. A group of muscles over the loins and croup are affected, accompanied by pain, lameness and disinclination to move. The muscles are rigid and the affected horse, when forced to move, does so with great difficulty. Other symptoms are rapid respiration, dilated nostrils, profuse sweating and sometimes the passing of coffee-coloured urine. The latter is not as consistent as in azoturia. When forced to walk, affected horses improve and often recover quickly, in contrast to the collapse and paralysis which occurs when cases of azoturia are exercised. The mortality rate is negligible and most affected animals make an uneventful recovery.

Treatment

Lack of basic knowledge as to the cause of the condition makes treatment difficult, but latest research work indicates the possible value of selenium and vitamin E in the treatment and prevention of the disease. Various drugs are used by veterinarians in symptomatic treatment and include preparations which produce relaxation. Sedatives, such as chloral hydrate, and tranquillizers are also used.

Pending the arrival of the veterinary surgeon, the horse should be well rubbed down, rugged if necessary, and quietly walked about with periodic rests. Hot fomentations over the muscles and gentle massage are of value.

NAVEL-ILL
See *Joint-ill*

NAVICULAR DISEASE
NAVICULAR disease is a chonic inflammation of a small shuttle-shaped bone and its associated structures within the foot.

The navicular bone rests against the back of the central part of the *os pedis* (coffin bone). The bone above (*os coronae*), sometimes referred to as the coronet bone, articulates with the coffin bone and the navicular bone, and rocks to and fro as the foot is moved. The navicular bone is covered with cartilage and the deep flexor tendon of the foot plays over it.

The disease is more common in light horses, being seldom seen in heavy breeds, and is almost invariably confined to the fore feet. It might be regarded as a chronic ostitis (inflammation of bone) with roughening of the articular cartilage and changes in the bone, which may lead to deformity and very occasionally, fracture of the bone. The disease often begins as a *bursitis* (inflammation of a bursa or small sac interposed between movable parts), affecting the navicular bursa, followed by adhesions between the bone and the deep flexor tendon.

Cause

The causes of the disease, other than a direct injury, are not definitely known. A number of theories have been advanced as to how the disease originates. Some of the suggested causes are: severe and continuous concussion on hard ground; compression of the navicular bone between the *os pedis* and the *os coronae* in front and the tendon behind, as may result from long standing in one position; hereditary predisposition; conformation, and faulty shoeing.

Symptoms

The symptoms of navicular disease usually develop slowly. An early symptom is "pointing" of the fore foot when the horse is standing at rest. The foot is placed in a position slightly in advance of the other fore foot, with the heel only just touching the ground. When both fore feet are affected, each is alternately pointed. Whilst "pointing" is a common symptom, it is not absolutely characteristic of navicular disease, because "pointing" may be shown in other painful conditions below the fetlock. Slight lameness is shown early in the course of the disease. The horse may take a few lame steps or appear stiff when first worked in the morning, but the lameness then disappears. Alternatively, it may start off sound and become lame during the day. The stride is shortened and there is a tendency to stumble. The lameness is more likely to be shown on hard ground and when the horse is turned in a short circle.

The following day the horse may appear to be quite sound. This intermittent lameness persists for some time but eventually lameness becomes more constant. Pain may be evident by pressing with the thumb in the hollow of the heel or by firm pressure on the frog with a pair of farrier's pincers. The gait is altered; changes in the form of the foot become evident, due to the fact that the horse continually saves the heels, and in due course the horse becomes unfit for work.

Treatment

Few cases of navicular disease recover. Treatment generally only alleviates the condition but does not result in a cure. The horse must be rested. The foot should receive attention by thinning the quarters with a rasp to relieve pressure where the foot is contracted; by shortening the toe; paring the sole, and leaving the heels alone. The

129

horse may now be shod with rolled-toe or half-round shoes and heel calkins. The latter relieve tension on the deep flexor tendon. A veterinarian with the assistance of a good farrier can accomplish a good deal to keep the horse in working condition for some time. Finally, the operation of neurectomy (cutting a portion of a nerve) will give relief from pain and prolong the usefulness of the animal for light work.

NETTLE RASH (Urticaria, Hives)

THIS is an allergic condition characterized by the sudden appearance of a number of rounded, elevated areas in the skin over the head and neck or on the body.

Cause

Urticaria occurs when sensitive animals develop an allergic reaction after eating certain foods, or as a result of insect stings or from contact with the stinging nettle (hence the more common name), or other stinging plants. Similar elevated areas of the skin are sometimes seen in association with some specific diseases such as strangles and influenza.

Symptoms

Usually the only symptoms observed are the rapid appearance of the swellings in the skin on various parts of the body, which vary in size from ¼ to 2 inches in diameter. Sometimes they are larger. The swellings have a flat top, are tense to the touch and no exudate or weeping occurs. There is little or no itching except with insect or plant stings. It is common for the swellings to subside in a few hours, but the condition may persist on the horse for 3 or 4 days, apparently due to the appearance of fresh lesions. There may be slight constitutional upset, as shown by irregular bowel movement.

Treatment

The skin eruption commonly clears up without treatment, especially if the feed is changed or the animal is removed from pasture where nettles and other stinging plants occur, or the horse can be protected from stinging insects. The subcutaneous injection of antihistamine drugs, which are readily available, is the best form of treatment. When irritation is shown, cooling astringent lotions, such as calamine lotion, white lotion or a dilute solution of sodium bicarbonate (baking soda) can be used to advantage. A mild purgative should be given followed by a few bran mashes and change of diet.

NURSING A SICK HORSE

ALTHOUGH the sulphonamide and antibiotic drugs have greatly contributed to the treatment of disease, good nursing still plays an important part in restoring a horse to health and should not be neglected, as it is a valuable adjunct to the use of modern drugs. Without detracting from the importance of skilled veterinary attention, it can be said that many a horse has been saved by the good nursing of an attentive groom or owner.

The comfort of the patient is very important. Horses affected with certain respiratory diseases, such as pneumonia, will not lie down because they can breathe better standing up. Under these circumstances, bandaging the legs below the knees and hocks with Newmarket bandages gives leg support and warmth, which adds to the comfort of the animal. The bandages should be removed twice a day and the legs well rubbed before re-adjusting.

An unstabled horse should be placed in a fresh clean grass paddock, well protected from prevailing winds and, if the weather is cold, it should be lightly rugged by day and more heavily rugged at night. Water should be readily available. If the horse is accustomed to being stabled, it should for preference be placed in a loose-box or shed away from other horses, well bedded-down with straw, and disturbed as little as possible. Good ventilation without draughts is essential, fresh water should be provided, and rock-salt be available in the manger.

With few exceptions, illnesses are accompanied by a rise in temperature and a tendency to constipation. The horse is consequently disinclined to eat, and invalid foods of a laxative nature, such as a well-prepared bran mash, are called for. Instructions for the preparation of this mash are given under *Bran Mash*. It is necessary that the bran mash be freshly prepared and if it is found that the horse has not eaten it all, the remainder should be discarded, the manger or box thoroughly cleaned and a fresh mash prepared. The object is to tempt the horse to eat to keep up its strength and, if possible, to overcome constipation without drenching. In any case, purgative drenches should not be administered if a horse is affected with a sore throat or some respiratory complaint.

Freshly-cut green feed is usually attractive to a stabled horse. Other light, nourishing feeds which are easily prepared and which should be fed fresh, and in small quantities and often, are:

Oatmeal gruel prepared by mixing 1 lb. of oatmeal with a little
    water to form a paste and then adding this, with a little salt, to
    1 gallon of water and heating, stirring continuously until it boils,

after which it should be allowed to simmer until it is of uniform thickness. Many horses will eat this in preference to a more sloppy mixture.

Linseed tea prepared by boiling slowly ½ lb. of linseed in a gallon of water, and stirring repeatedly, until the grains are quite soft and it becomes the consistency of jelly. This is a very valuable article of diet for a sick horse, ½ to 1 lb. being added daily to other feed.

Hay tea prepared by filling a thoroughly clean bucket with long sweet hay, pouring boiling water over it and covering with a clean sack. Allow to stand until cold, and strain. This makes a refreshing drink for a sick horse and, although it does not contain much nourishment, is nevertheless of value.

Scalded oats prepared by pouring boiling water over 2 to 3 lb. of crushed oats in a clean bucket, adding a little salt and allowing to stand for fifteen minutes. This may be fed in small quantities or added to bran mashes.

When a horse is convalescent and concentrated foods are required to build up its strength, milk and eggs can be used to advantage. 6 eggs may be beaten up in a ½ gallon of whole or separated milk, a little salt added and the horse at first drenched with this until he has acquired the taste, when he may drink it from a bucket. Eggs may be boiled hard, cut up finely and fed with other tempting food, such as crumbled bread or broken biscuits. This is also a change from wet food, of which horses soon tire.

A sick horse should not be worried by the routine of grooming. Nevertheless wisping, hand-rubbing, and sponging the eyes, nostrils and dock contribute to the animal's comfort.

OPHTHALMIA

See *Eye—Conjunctivitis*, *Eye—Keratitis*, and *Eye—Periodic Ophthalmia*

PARALYSIS

BROADLY, paralysis means loss of nerve control over any of the bodily functions, but the term is usually used to describe loss of muscle function or of sensation, caused by injury to nerves or other interference with the nervous system.

Paralytic affections are of two kinds, the complete and the incomplete. The former include those in which both motion and sensibility are affected; the latter, those in which only one or other is lost or diminished. Paralysis may be general or partial. When only a small portion of the body is affected, such as the face, a limb or the tail, it is referred to as local paralysis.

Causes

These are varied. Most of the acute affections of the brain and spinal cord may lead to paralysis. Injuries, tumours and disease of the blood vessels of the brain (including the so-called redworms or bloodworms in the blood vessels), are some of the causes of paralysis. Pressure upon, or the severing of a nerve causes a paralysis of the parts to which such a nerve is distributed. Apoplexy may be termed a general paralysis and in non-fatal cases, is a frequent cause of the various forms of paralysis.

Treatment

In view of the fact that there are so many causes and different types of paralysis, professional aid should be obtained as soon as possible. Until such assistance is available, the horse should be kept quiet and, if necessary, secured in such a way that it cannot suffer serious injury from accidents.

PARASITES—INTERNAL

THE HORSE harbours a variety of internal parasites, some more harmful than others. Probably no individual animal is ever entirely free of some of them but, unless heavy infection occurs, the less important species do no real damage to the horse, especially if it is well fed and kept under good conditions. On the other hand, certain parasites can be extremely harmful and be responsible for death of the animal. The majority of worm parasites of the horse develop in the digestive tract, although some of them, such as the so-called redworms or bloodworms, spend part of their life history in other parts of the body.

Infection with internal parasites can be responsible for such common troubles as poor condition, rapid tiring when working and digestive disturbances. There are few horse-owners who have not had some first-hand experience with worms in horses, but considerable misunderstanding exists as to the damage done by the various types of parasites. The commonest misunderstanding is to attribute the poor condition of the horse to the larger parasites which can be readily seen in the droppings or at a post-mortem examination, whereas the trouble is more likely to be due to other very small parasites which are less readily recognized.

A complete classification of horse parasites is not justified here, nor would it be very helpful to the horse-owner. The commonest parasites of the horse in this country are the redworms or blood-worms, large roundworm, stomach worms, pinworms, tapeworms and the larval stage of the bot fly. The latter parasite has been dealt with under *Bots*. Of the parasites listed, those that are responsible for the greatest amount of ill-health in horses and which not infrequently cause death are the redworms, especially in foals. Next in importance is the large roundworm.

REDWORMS OR BLOODWORMS

There are several varieties of the so-called redworm or bloodworm which have the common generic name of *Strongylus*. Their life histories and the effect they have on the horse are similar. The mature worms are from a half to two inches in length and about the thickness of the lead in an ordinary pencil. The colour is whitish-brown if free in the bowel, but red if they have sucked blood, hence the common names. Infective larvae are picked up and swallowed by

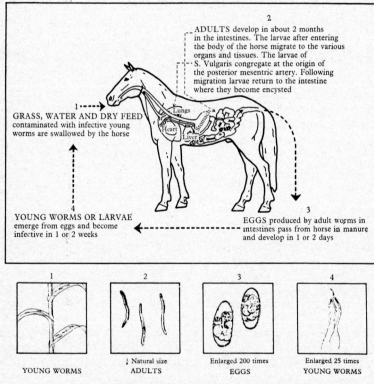

Fig. 55 Life History of Red Worm, *Strongylus vulgaris*.
(*F. Thorp and R. Graham, University of Illinois, College of Agriculture*)

134

the horse when grazing. After casting off their protective skins, the larvae burrow into the wall of the bowel, enter the bloodstream and are then carried to the liver, lungs and elsewhere. The larvae may enter the walls of the arteries, causing much damage and large blood clots. After some months, the worms migrate back to the bowel wall and wander through and into the bowel, eventually becoming adults, male and female, seven to eight months after the larvae were swallowed. Large numbers of eggs are laid in the bowel and passed out in the droppings.

The wandering immature redworms, particularly those of *Strongylus vulgaris*, damage liver, lungs and bowel wall. While in the blood vessels, the worms cause aneurysms (obstructive swellings) which may interfere with the supply of blood to the intestines, resulting in digestive upsets and attacks of colic. Sometimes the wall of the blood vessel becomes so weakened by the activities of the worms that it ruptures and the horse dies of internal haemorrhage. When the arteries supplying blood to the hind legs are affected, a horse may sway and even fall when doing hard work.

Adult worms feed on the lining of the bowel and large numbers cause loss of blood, irritation to the bowel, indigestion, intermittent diarrhoea, constipation and even rupture of the bowel.

Horses of all ages are subject to the ravages of redworms, foals becoming infected as soon as they commence to graze.

Treatment

A number of drugs have been found to be effective against Strongyles including thiabendazole, sold under the proprietary name of *Thibenzole*; phenothiazine and piperazine compounds. *Thibenzole* can be recommended as safe and highly effective against redworms. The preparation can be purchased in powder form in 4 oz. packets. The dose rate is ¼ oz. of dry powder per 250 lb. of body weight, that is 1 oz. for a 1,000 lb. horse. The powder may be fed well mixed in the feed. It is also available as a liquid preparation, the dose rate of which is half a fluid ounce per 100 lb. body weight, that is five fluid ounces for a 1,000 lb. horse. Starvation before treatment is not necessary. Full directions are given on the containers.

Prevention

Avoid overstocking of paddocks with horses and adopt rotational grazing if possible. Other stock may be run in the paddock being spelled, as the redworms only infect horses.

Yards and stables should be kept free of droppings and particular attention should be directed to the protection of foals by treating the mares before the foals are born, to reduce the risk of them

135

becoming infected from the pasture soon after birth. If a number of horses are run on a property, or horse breeding is carried out, an organized plan of campaign should be adopted to minimize the harmful effects of these serious parasites. Such a campaign is best carried out under the supervision of a veterinarian.

THE LARGE ROUNDWORM

The common large roundworm, *Ascaris (Parascaris) equorum*, which infects the horse is quite a large worm, measuring from six to fourteen inches in length and half an inch in diameter. It resembles an earthworm in shape, is yellowish-white in colour and is commonly seen in the droppings of infected horses. It does not do as much harm as redworms, which are not so commonly seen, but can be very troublesome in foals.

The adult worms live mainly in the small bowel, where the females lay large numbers of eggs which are passed out in the droppings. These do not hatch on the ground and become infective larvae, as in the case of the redworms. In ten to fourteen days the larvae

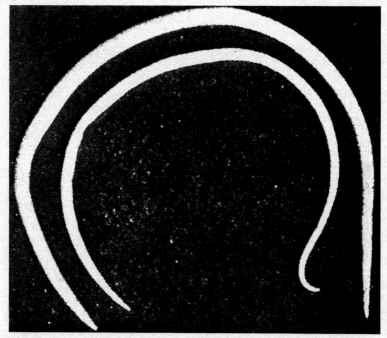

Fig. 56 The Large Roundworm Parascaris equorum (two-thirds natural size).
(*Illinois College of Agriculture*)

136

develop inside the eggs which are subsequently picked up by the horse when grazing or licked up by the foal in the stable or yard. In the intestine, the egg covering dissolves and the larvae emerge and burrow into the wall of the intestine, enter the bloodstream and are carried to the liver. Here they feed and grow and subsequently re-enter the bloodstream and are carried to the lungs. The larvae later enter the air passages of the lungs and are coughed up into the throat and swallowed back into the stomach. They pass on to the small intestine, where they grow rapidly. At the end of ten weeks, they are mature and the females start laying eggs, thus starting the life cycle again. The whole life cycle inside the horse takes two to three months to complete. The eggs may survive many months on pasture and in stables.

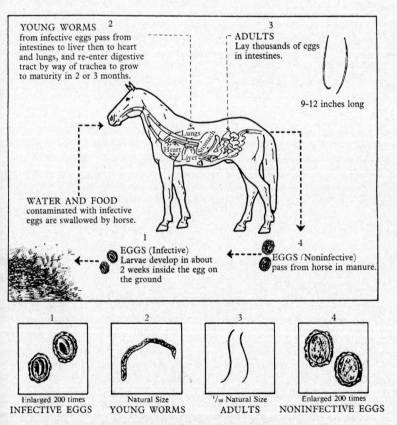

Fig. 57   The Life History of Large Roundworm, *Parascaris equorum.*
(*F. Thorp and R. Graham, University of Illinois, College of Agriculture*)

Harmful Effects

Young horses up to two years of age and especially foals, suffer most from roundworm infection. Older horses seem to develop a resistance to the parasite. Bronchitis and even pneumonia occur in foals as a result of the migration of the immature roundworms to the lungs. This would depend largely on the extent of the infection. Later, as the adult worms develop in the small intestine, unthriftiness, stunted growth, harsh coat, scouring, rapid tiring and digestive trouble result. These parasites are sometimes so numerous that they block up the small intestine and give rise to colic which may kill the animal. They occasionally cause perforation of the bowel, resulting in fatal peritonitis.

Treatment

For many years, carbon bisulphide has been widely used for the removal of large roundworms from horses and has the additional advantage that it is also effective against the larvae of the bot fly ("bots") in the stomach of the horse. The drug must be administered expertly in a gelatine capsule or by stomach tube, and therefore its use usually requires the services of a veterinarian. The dose rate is 5 ml. per 100 lb. body weight. Dose for foals (8 weeks) 10 ml., yearlings 10 to 15 ml., adults 20 ml. The horse should be starved, but given access to water, for 18 to 24 hours before giving the drug, and for four hours afterwards. The treatment should not be followed by a purgative drench. Piperazine compounds have also been found very effective against roundworms but their use should be left to a veterinarian. There are other treatments, and some effective new drugs such as *Neguvon* can be used under veterinary supervision.

Prevention

It is very difficult to prevent foals and other horses from becoming infected with roundworms, because the female worm produces enormous numbers of eggs which are scattered far and wide in the droppings. The objective is to keep the contamination rate as low as possible by killing the worms in young horses and adopting methods of management to reduce the possibility of infection. If brood mares are infected, they should be treated before foaling, which should take place in paddocks which have been spelled or upon which stock other than horses have been running. Overstocking of paddocks with horses should be avoided. Stables should be cleaned out daily and yards kept free of droppings. Manure disposal is important. It should be piled in a heap and covered so that the heat generated during fermentation of the manure will kill most of the roundworm eggs. This is also effective in killing the infective larvae of the redworms.

STOMACH WORMS

In addition to the larva of the bot fly which infects the stomach of the horse and which is discussed under "Bots", there are found in the stomach several species of worms which give rise to gastritis and digestive disorder.

THE SMALL STOMACH WORM (*Trichostrongylus axei*)

This worm is not of great importance in Australia. It is a very small worm, a quarter to half an inch long and hair-like, and is similar to the fine hair worm seen in sheep and cattle. The mode of development is broadly similar to other worms of this type, except that it does not wander in the body of the animal. These worms are too small to be readily seen, but infection can frequently be diagnosed at post-mortem examination by the appearance of a number of isolated, raised, button-like areas on the lining membrane of the stomach. Heavy infections with these parasites can cause rapid loss of condition in the horse.

LARGE STOMACH WORM (*Habronema spp.*)

The most troublesome worms infecting the stomach of the horse are the so-called large stomach worms of the *Habronema* species. Actually, there are three species of this type of worm which infect horses in Australia. They are all slender white worms measuring one-half to one and a quarter inches in length. The life history is quite different to the life histories of the worms already described. The adult female lays its eggs in the stomach of the horse and these eggs are passed out in the droppings. For further development to take place, these eggs must be swallowed within about eight days by the maggots of house flies, stable flies or other flies that breed in horse manure. Within the fly maggot, a larva develops from the egg, but does not undergo complete development until the fly matures. The fully developed larva is now found in the proboscis (snout) of the fly, from where it infects the horse when the fly is feeding around the mouth or elsewhere on the head of the horse. Those larvae which are swallowed by the horse reach the stomach where they develop to maturity, egg-laying takes place, and the cycle starts over again.

Harmful Effects

The large stomach worm can cause more than one type of trouble. Those larvae which are swallowed by the horse generally live close to the glands of the stomach, embedded in mucus. Some species burrow deep into the stomach wall and, as a result of bacterial infection, abscesses are formed which have the appearance of tumour-

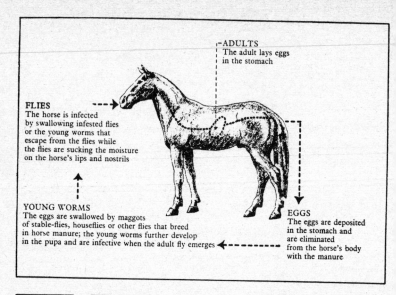

FLIES
The horse is infected
by swallowing infested flies
or the young worms that
escape from the flies while
the flies are sucking the moisture
on the horse's lips and nostrils

ADULTS
The adult lays eggs
in the stomach

YOUNG WORMS
The eggs are swallowed by maggots
of stable-flies, houseflies or other flies that breed
in horse manure; the young worms further develop
in the pupa and are infective when the adult fly emerges

EGGS
The eggs are deposited
in the stomach and
are eliminated
from the horse's body
with the manure

A-ADULTS
⅓ Natural size

B-EGGS
Enlarged 150 times

STOMACH WORMS

A-MAGGOT
Enlarged 2 times

B-PUPA
Enlarged 4 times

C-ADULT
Enlarged 4 times

FLY CARRIERS

Fig. 58 Life History of Large Stomach Worm, *Habronema spp.*
(*F. Thorp and R. Graham, University of Illinois, College of Agriculture*)

like masses on the wall of the stomach. Although these abscesses occasionally cause acute conditions, such as haemorrhage and perforation of the stomach, generally they are responsible for irritation and damage to the glandular mucous membrane of the stomach with resultant digestive upset, and possibly colic.

On the other hand, those larvae that are deposited by the fly around the corner of the eye of the horse or in small wounds and scratches on the body, produce the condition commonly referred to as "summer sores" or habronema granuloma. These conditions are produced by the larvae burrowing into the tissues and irritating them, sometimes causing granulation tissue or proud flesh to form. In the corner of the eye, this granulation tissue has the appearance of a growth and is frequently mistaken for cancer of the eye. Similar effects may occur on other parts of the body wherever there are moist conditions which attract the fly, such as the sheath of a horse, wound surfaces and even the pasterns and fetlocks.

Treatment

Some degree of success can be obtained in the treatment of the small stomach worm by drenching with carbon tetrachloride in paraffin or raw linseed oil after 24 hours starvation. The dose is 10 ml. of carbon tetrachloride per 100 lb. body weight. The dose for heavy draughts is 50 ml., light draughts 40 ml., thoroughbred types 30 ml., ponies 20 to 25 ml. The drug is mixed with about a pint of one of the oils mentioned and given as a drench. It is preferable to administer it by a stomach tube.

The treatment of large stomach worms (*Habronema spp.*) involves washing out the stomach with bicarbonate of soda solution by means of a stomach tube, and then administering carbon bisulphide by stomach tube. This treatment should only be carried out by a veterinary surgeon. A complex compound known as *Safersan*, which releases carbon bisulphide in the stomach, has been found very effective against *Habronema spp.* It should also be administered by a veterinarian.

Prevention

The control of the small stomach worm is along the lines of good stable and yard hygiene, involving constant disposal of manure in the manner already described, the avoidance of overstocking of horse paddocks, and routine treatment where necessary.

In the case of the large stomach worm (*Habronema spp.*), the same general considerations apply regarding hygiene but it is also important to break the life cycle by preventing flies from breeding and by destroying them. This can be done by the effective disposal of manure by piling it in heaps and covering it so that the heat generated will destroy the parasitic eggs or fly larvae, or by placing the manure in fly-proof pits. In and around the stables and yards, flies may be destroyed by regular spraying with an effective residual insecticide during the summer months.

PINWORMS

The pinworm (*Oxyuris equi*) is a slender, whitish, thread-like worm, commonly seen around the anus of the horse. The female pinworm measures up to six inches in length and has a fine pointed tail. The male is very small, about an inch in length. Actually pinworms do not do a great deal of harm and only rarely do heavy infections lead to loss of condition.

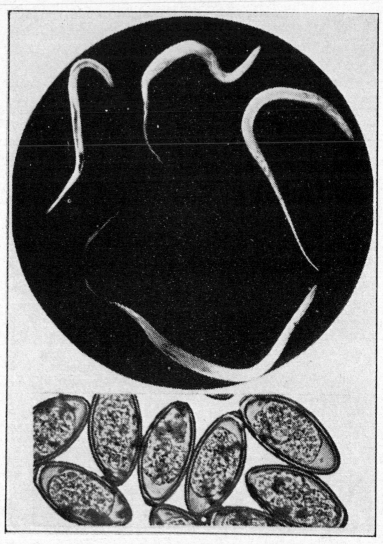

Fig. 59 Pinworms, *Oxyuris equi*, and Eggs. Mature worms ⅔ natural size; the eggs are greatly enlarged.

(*F. Thorp and R. Graham, University of Illinois, College of Agriculture*)

The immature forms of these worms inhabit the caecum and large colon of the horse, where they develop without migration elsewhere in the body. The mature female wanders down or is carried with the dung to the rectum and does not normally leave the body completely, but at intervals wriggles partly out of the anus and deposits eggs, together with a sticky material. This enables the eggs to adhere in clusters to the skin around and below the anus. When egg laying is complete, the female dies. Development within the egg is rapid. In 24 to 36 hours a motile larva is present, and the eggs are infective in three days. The eggs are rubbed off or drop to the ground, where they are later picked up by horses when grazing.

Harmful Effects

Due to the irritation caused by the sticky material surrounding the eggs, the horse rubs its hindquarters against posts and fences, thus removing the hair from the tail. Close examination will reveal the egg masses around the anus.

Treatment

The skin around the anus may be smeared with white mercuric or carbolic ointment. Anthelmintic medication may be carried out if necessary. Piperazine compounds and *Thibenzole* have been found to be effective.

Prevention

Thorough daily grooming will remove eggs from the anal region before they become infective.

TAPEWORMS

Tapeworms do occur in the horse but they are not common, nor are they of much importance. These worms are flat, segmented and vary according to the species from one inch to 12 inches in length and up to half an inch in width. They are found in the small intestine. As the worms mature, segments containing eggs are shed and passed in the droppings where they are sometimes seen. The intermediate host is a small mite found on pastures, which is ingested by the horse when feeding. The damage caused by tapeworms in horses is so slight that treatment is not warranted. Regular treatment against other internal parasites will offset any damage likely to be done by tapeworms.

PARTURITION

MARES in this country are usually allowed to foal in a clean, well-grassed paddock in which there is adequate shelter and a plentiful water supply. It is best that the mare be left alone and disturbed as

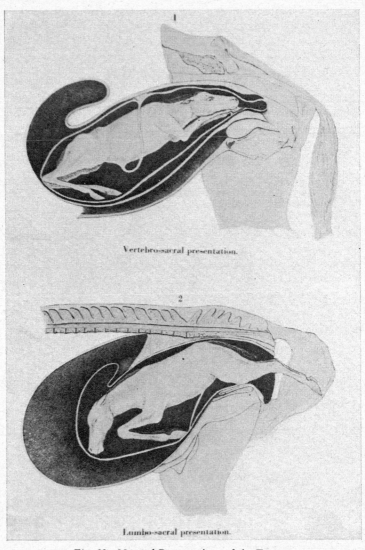

Vertebro-sacral presentation.

Lumbo-sacral presentation.

Fig. 60 Normal Presentations of the Foetus.

(*From Diseases of the Horse.
United States Department of Agriculture*)

144

little as possible, whilst at the same time keeping her under close observation.

The signs of approaching parturition include a gradual enlargement of the udder about three to six weeks before foaling. A sticky secretion oozes away from the teats as long as eight to ten days before the birth, but sometimes not until close to foaling. This forms a wax-like coating around the teat openings (waxing-up). The belly drops, the flanks fall in and the loins may become depressed. Swelling of the vulva is noted, which increases as foaling approaches. Finally, the mare becomes uneasy, has an anxious look, stops feeding, switches and elevates the tail, strains and may lie down and get up again several times. As the time of parturition approaches, the lips of the swollen vulva swell out and a copious slimy discharge is shown. There may be considerable variation in the periods at which some of the above signs are shown.

The Act of Foaling

The mare frequently foals when she is down. In other cases, the act is accomplished standing. Violent contractions of the womb and abdominal muscles take place and the "water bags" appear and burst, followed normally by the fore feet of the foal, with the nose between them, and then, after a few more expulsive efforts of the mare, the foal is expelled. The whole act may be over in five to ten minutes. The navel cord, which connects the foal to the membranes, is ruptured when the foal falls to the ground, or when the mare rises if she has been down. The afterbirth comes away shortly afterwards, but may be delayed from three to six hours. This should be disposed of by burial or burning. Mares that have foaled should receive a properly prepared bran mash daily for three days, in order that the bowels will be kept loose and constipation avoided. Thereafter, they may be placed on their normal diet.

The stump of the navel cord of the foal may be dusted with sulphanilamide powder or treated with some mild antiseptic, but must not be tied.

Natural Presentation

With natural presentations, there is rarely any difficulty at parturition. When there is a single foal, the natural presentation is with the fore feet first, the nose between the knees, and with the front of the hoofs and knees and the forehead directed upwards. In this way the natural curvature of the body of the foetus corresponds to the curve of the womb and genital passages, particularly of the bony pelvis, and so the foal passes out easily. When there is a twin birth, the second foal usually comes with the hind feet first, and the back of the legs,

145

the points of the hocks and the tail and croup turned upwards. In this presentation, the curvature of the body of the foal still corresponds to that of the passage, and its expulsion may be just as easy. Any presentations apart from these two may be said to be abnormal and may result in a difficult birth.

Difficult Parturition

There are many causes of difficult birth. Sometimes birth commences before relaxation of the pelvis and dilation of the cervix. Narrowness of the pelvic outlet can be a problem, particularly in underdeveloped mares, or there may be mechanical obstruction due to overweight, pressure of tumours, constipation or abnormal conformation.

Sometimes the foal may be presented in an abnormal position. Some of the common types of abnormal presentations are forelegs presented and the head deflected; head and one foreleg presented and the other foreleg under the body; head presented and knees bent; one foreleg presented with head and other foreleg bent back; both forelegs presented and head down; knees bent and head under chest; foal on its back with head and forelegs pointing backwards; four legs and head presented. There are many other abnormal presentations.

Although most mares foal normally and rapidly, difficult and delayed presentations are serious and require skill and care in handling. Whereas a layman can often overcome some cases of difficult parturition in a cow, similar assistance given to a mare is likely to be disastrous. Difficult parturition in a mare is a matter for a qualified veterinary surgeon. In an emergency, and should professional assistance not be available, an attempt might be made to rectify a minor abnormal presentation. The greatest cleanliness must be observed. The whole arm and hand of the operator should be thoroughly washed with soap and warm water and then smeared with petroleum jelly. The nails must be cut short. The hand should be inserted with the thumb and fingers drawn together in the form of a cone. Whether lying or standing, the head of the mare should be downhill, and the hindparts raised as much as possible. This facilitates the exploratory examination and manipulations. Any traction should always be downwards towards the mare's hocks, pulling when she strains and resting when she rests.

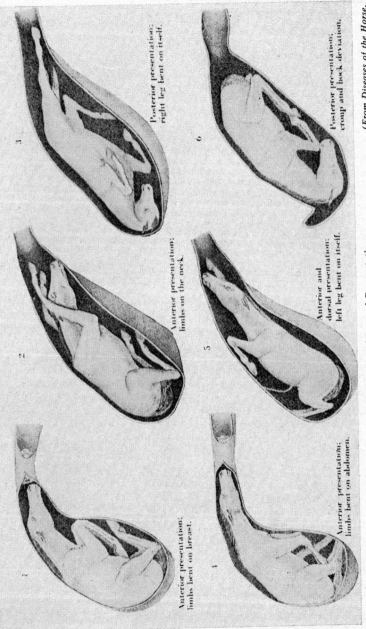

Anterior presentation: limbs bent on breast.

Anterior presentation: limbs on the neck.

Posterior presentation: right leg bent on itself.

Anterior presentation: limbs bent on abdomen.

Anterior and dorsal presentation: left leg bent on itself.

Posterior presentation: croup and back deviation.

Fig. 61 Abnormal Presentations.

(From Diseases of the Horse.
United States Department of Agriculture)

147

L

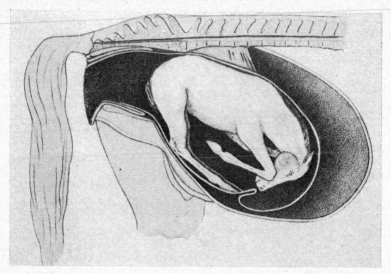

Fig. 62   Abnormal Presentation. Thigh and Croup presentation.
*(From Diseases of the Horse.
United States Department of Agriculture)*

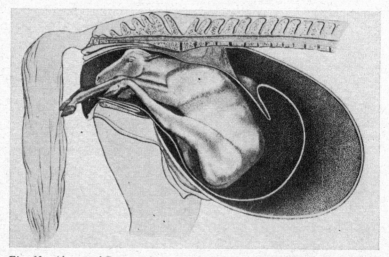

Fig. 63   Abnormal Presentation. Anterior presentation. Hind limb deviation.
*(From Diseases of the Horse.
United States Department of Agriculture)*

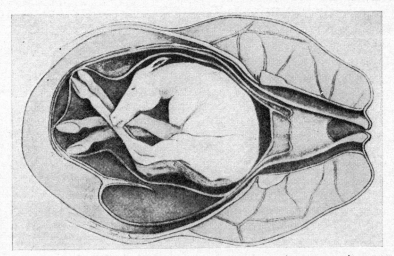

Fig. 64   Abnormal Presentation. Transverse presentation—upper view.

(From Diseases of the Horse.
United States Department of Agriculture)

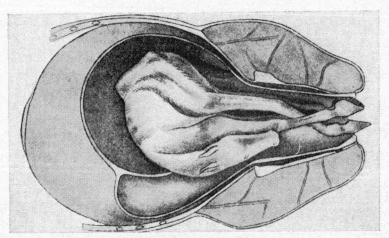

Fig. 65   Abnormal Presentation. Sterno-abdominal presentation—head and feet engaged.

(From Diseases of the Horse.
United States Department of Agriculture)

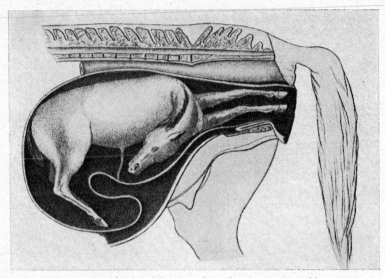

Fig. 66   Abnormal Presentation—head turned on side.

(From Diseases of the Horse.
United States Department of Agriculture)

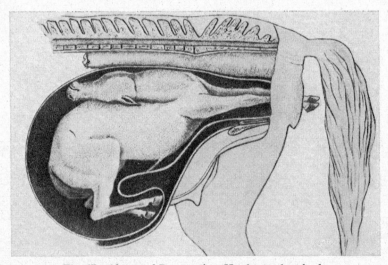

Fig. 67   Abnormal Presentation. Head turned on back.

(From Diseases of the Horse.
United States Department of Agriculture)

PERVIOUS URACHUS ("Leaking Navel")

PERVIOUS urachus occurs in the newborn and is a fairly common condition in foals. Up to the time of birth, the urine is discharged through the urachus (a small ureter-like structure within the umbilical cord), into a membranous bag called the allantoic sac, one of the "water bags" surrounding the foetus. In this way, it is prevented from entering the inner "water bag", the amniotic sac, where it would mingle with the liquids directly surrounding the foetus and cause irritation. This structure usually closes when the umbilical cord is ruptured at birth, and the urine takes the normal course and is voided through the bladder and urethra. It sometimes happens that the closure of the urachus is imperfect and a continuous dribbling of urine from the region of the umbilicus of the young foal keeps the area wet, although, in addition, urine may still be passed in the natural way.

This is not a very serious condition and is readily treated by a veterinarian, but if the leaking persists for any great length of time, the moist condition around the umbilicus favours bacterial infection of the navel stump, leading to joint-ill and other troubles.

Treatment

Most cases will correct themselves within a few days, but it is undesirable to delay treatment longer than this, when a veterinarian should be called in to cauterize the urachus. The navel cord must not be tied to correct this condition. More serious cases, especially when the entire contents of the bladder are being passed through the urachus, will require surgical intervention.

PERIOSTITIS

PERIOSTITIS means inflammation of the surface of the bone and its covering membrane, the periosteum. The condition is commonly known in racing stables as "sore shins". It may be followed by inflammation of the bone itself (*ostitis*), which shows as a roughened bony surface generally to the front of the cannon bone. Sore shins are usually seen in the forelegs, particularly in young racehorses in training, and are due to concussion. The more severe forms are associated with bacterial activity.

Symptoms

The horse walks in a sore and tender manner, especially after a gallop on hard ground. Signs of inflammation, as shown by soreness, may be obscure at first, but later there is a soft fluctuating swelling which eventually becomes hard. During the early stages, the swelling is painful to the touch; the horse keeps shifting its feet if both legs are affected, or points the toe and bends the fetlock joint if the trouble is only in one leg. In very severe cases, where the bone tissue has become infected, there is a rise in temperature, the horse goes off its food, is disinclined to move and is lame.

Treatment

Cold applications either by hosing or the application of ice poultices, followed by warm applications and hand rubbing, are usually sufficient to cut short mild attacks. *Antiphlogistine* applied under a light bandage is useful. The horse should be rested from work, but may be given light exercise on soft ground. A laxative diet is desirable. In more severe cases, iodine ointment may be used or a light blister may be necessary. If a blister is applied, the usual precautions must be taken to tie the horse up short to prevent it biting the leg, and petroleum jelly used to prevent the blister running. When bone is infected, antibiotic injections will be necessary. The horse must be brought back into work gradually, exercising at first on soft ground only.

PERITONITIS

PERITONITIS means inflammation of the serous membrane lining the cavity of the abdomen and covering the organs. It is most frequently caused by injuries, such as punctured wounds of the abdomen, severe blows or kicks and sometimes occurs following the operation of castration, or an operation for hernia. Peritonitis can also occur during the course of certain infectious diseases.

Symptoms

These include fever, distress, disinclination to move, stiffness of the abdominal walls, which are painful when touched; frequent passage of small quantities of urine with pain; attempts to lie down with bending of knees and hocks but failure to carry out the intention. Constipation is usually present and may be followed by scouring. There is a rapid pulse and the visible mucous membranes, such as those of the eyes and the nose, are congested. If death does not occur within a few days, an extensive effusion of fluid occurs in the abdominal cavity leading to a condition known as ascites or dropsy, and the abdomen is distended.

Treatment

The services of a veterinarian are required to administer wide-spectrum antibiotics and probably also sulphonamides systemically. If perforation of the abdomen has occurred, corrective surgery will be necessary. If professional assistance is not available, hot fomentations by blankets around the belly and the use of counter-irritants over the belly, such as mustard plasters, may be of some value. Any punctured wound should receive appropriate treatment by thorough cleansing and the use of some mild antiseptic solution and then dusting with sulphanilamide powder. Purgative drenches should not be given, but 1 oz. of chloral hydrate in a quart of water or, for preference, in thin gruel can be given to relieve pain. The mortality rate from peritonitis is very high in the horse.

PHOTOSENSITIZATION (Trefoil Dermatitis)

PHOTOSENSITIZATION develops when the animal is in a state of photosensitivity due to the presence in the bloodstream of certain photodynamic or sensitizing substances of plant or chemical origin. These predispose the unpigmented skin to the harmful effects of ultra-violet rays. On rare occasions even pigmented skin is affected. Plants capable of producing light sensitization are referred to as photodynamic plants.

Horses are affected only with simple or primary photosensitization and apparently do not suffer from the type associated with damage to the liver as occurs in sheep. A dermatitis of the unpigmented areas of the skin of horses, without obvious liver damage, has been known for a long time following the eating of certain medicagos and trefoils such as *Trifolium pratense*, *T. hybridum*, *Medicago sativa* and *Medicago polymorpha*.

In the days when draught horses were used for farming, trefoil dermatitis was a fairly common condition on the white portions of the skin, but particularly on the white fetlocks and legs of Clydesdale horses, in seasons of luxuriant herbage growth and much bright sunlight. Because aphids were frequently present on the trefoil and these were also seen on the white legs of the horses, the disease was commonly referred to as "aphis disease". Whilst the work of many investigators has not shown any association between aphis infestation and the toxicity of the trefoil plants, scientists working on the pigments of aphids have found a photodynamic substance in the aphids, and it is now suggested that this agent may be absorbed from the aphids eaten with the plants, which may contribute in some way to the development of the disease.

Symptoms

The lesions of photosensitization in horses occur mainly on the white or unpigmented parts of the skin such as the legs, the nose and face and in piebald horses on the white portions of the neck and body. The skin on the unpigmented areas is at first red, becomes thickened owing to the presence of fluid in the deeper layers and fluid may ooze from the surface. Itching occurs and the parts often become covered with crusts or scabs of dried exudate and blood. Quite commonly, as a result of the animal biting or rubbing the affected parts against logs and fences, large, raw areas are produced. These may become dry and cracked, or, following secondary infection, exude pus. Dead, leathery skin may be shed in large flakes. In white-muzzled horses, lesions occurring about the mouth may interfere with feeding.

Treatment

On the first signs of photosensitization, horses should be removed to another pasture, free of trefoils and clovers and containing plenty of shade, the last being very important. If practicable, the horses should be stabled or shedded and hand-fed. Treatment will vary according to the severity and extent of the lesions. Zinc cream or calamine lotion may be used to relieve itching. Hard crusts may be softened and their removal facilitated by raw linseed oil and lime water (50-50). If the lesions have become infected, they should be treated as infected wounds—see *Wounds*.

When horses have to be left in the open, an attempt should be made to darken the unpigmented areas of the skin to give some protection from the sun. This may be done by mixing lamp black or soot with equal parts by weight of petroleum jelly and smearing this over the affected portions of the skin, and other unpigmented areas if practicable. A fairly strong solution of potassium permanganate (*Condy's crystals*) will also darken the skin. Unfortunately, most pigments do not last long. Internal treatment is of little value, but if the horse is stabled, a laxative drench may be given to advantage. Antihistamine injections may be of some use in early cases. With prompt treatment and good nursing, particularly in the shade, the lesions usually heal satisfactorily. Severe cases may need veterinary attention.

PLEURISY

PLEURISY or pleuritis is an inflammation of the serous membrane lining the chest cavity and enveloping the lungs. It is not a common disease in horses except for its association with pneumonia, and as a complication of influenza or strangles. It may also be caused by a penetrating injury through the chest wall or a rib fracture. The condition may be acute or chronic.

154

Symptoms

The symptoms of acute pleurisy usually commence suddenly and often the first indication of the disease is that the horse is disinclined to move or turn around due to pain in the chest. There may be shivering, moderate temperature, dullness, and loss of appetite. The animal often sweats, is uneasy and may show mild signs of colic. Pressure or tapping over the chest between the ribs induces pain. The horse is usually stiff and walks as though foundered. The breathing is abdominal, the chest hardly moving at all and inspiration is short and jerky, the expiration longer. These latter symptoms indicate pain in the chest due to friction between the dry, inflamed, pleural surfaces of the chest and the lung. Application of the ear to the chest wall over the sensitive area may detect a dry-friction murmur. The horse prefers to stand rather than lie down. There may be a short, suppressed cough. After a few days, when effusion occurs, the patient appears to improve. The temperature drops somewhat, the pain decreases and the horse eats a little. The friction sound disappears as the exudation in the chest cavity builds up, moistening the pleural surfaces. Percussion or tapping with the fingers on the chest reveals a horizontal line of dullness which gradually rises higher in the chest as the fluid accumulates. The course of the disease varies. In mild cases, the fluid undergoes absorption and the case may terminate favourably in a week to ten days, although some adhesions of the pleurae may remain. In the more severe cases, when the quantity of effusion is large, the process of absorption is retarded. Respirations now become more frequent and rapid and the horse has an anxious and haggard expression and gradually weakens. Swelling may appear under the chest, extending to the abdomen and even the legs. In unfavourable cases, particularly when the pleural fluid contains pus, death usually occurs in two or three weeks.

Recovered animals sometimes have permanent disability due to adhesions in the chest cavity, the bands of fibrous tissue causing embarrassment to the free movement of the lungs. Such cases become "short in their wind" and "grunters".

Treatment

Pleurisy does not respond well to home treatment, although good nursing and general care of the patient contribute greatly to recovery. Veterinary assistance should be obtained in order that appropriate sulphonamide and antibiotic treatment can be carried out early. When there is an excessive amount of fluid in the chest cavity threatening collapse of the lungs, it may be necessary to draw off part of this fluid by puncturing the chest cavity. This should be left to a veterinarian to perform. It usually has to be repeated. Supportive treatment, especially in the early stages when there is much pain, can include the use of mustard plasters or hot blankets applied to the chest.

PNEUMONIA

PNEUMONIA is an inflammation of the lung substance caused by various agents such as viruses, bacteria, parasites, fungi, or the aspiration of dust and other foreign substances into the lungs. It is commonly complicated by inflammation of the bronchioles and/or pleurisy, and occurs as a complication of a number of specific diseases. Predisposing causes include inclement weather, fatigue, poorly-ventilated stables and sheds, bad sanitation and transportation with associated fatigue and lowered resistance.

Aspiration pneumonia is caused most frequently by careless or incompetent drenching, such as raising the head too high, giving the drench too fast, or interfering with the throat region to make the horse swallow. Drenching a horse when it is suffering from laryngitis or other respiratory conditions, attempting to drench an animal when it is down, and passing a stomach tube into the windpipe instead of the gullet are other causes. The disease produced is a necrotic or gangrenous pneumonia and is usually fatal.

The various forms of pneumonia are not discussed, but the general symptoms of all types of the disease are given below.

Pneumonia in the horse, apart from aspiration pneumonia, occurs mainly in foals or young horses and in old and debilitated animals.

General Symptoms

These are rises in temperature, not uncommonly reaching 104 to 105° F.; increased pulse rate; rapid shallow respirations which are abdominal in character; cough; nasal discharge; loss of appetite and great depression. When the temperature is very high, the horse sweats profusely. The nostrils are inflamed and dilated, the mucous membranes of the eyes are red, and the horse stands with head stretched forward, appearing to be afraid to lie down, and usually remains standing. In the early stages of catarrhal pneumonia, if the ear is held close to the chest, or a stethoscope is used, a gurgling sound may be heard, due to the air being forced through inflammatory liquid in the air sacs. After 12 to 24 hours, listening over the same area will reveal no sound owing to consolidation of that portion of the lung.

The course of primary, acute pneumonia varies, but in the horse it is usually less than a week after which, if the animal is going to recover, the general symptoms described above subside, the cough becomes loose and the appetite returns. If improvement does not occur within the first week, the prognosis is poor and death is likely.

Some cases continue as a chronic pneumonia and make a partial recovery. With early diagnosis, prompt and correct treatment and good nursing, the prognosis is more favourable.

Treatment

Sulphonamide and antibiotic drugs are now the routine treatment for all types of pneumonia. They should be administered by or under the supervision of a veterinarian. The choice of the antibiotic and its use in combination with a mixture of sulphonamides can be very important in the successful treatment of the animal. It is necessary that the drugs provide a wide spectrum of action against the potential infectious agents. Treatment with these drugs is necessary until the temperature has been normal for 24 hours. This usually entails a four-day course of treatment. Stimulating drugs can also be administered subcutaneously.

Supportive treatment combined with good nursing should not be neglected. Warmth and protection from adverse weather conditions are necessary for the patient, but in favourable weather an unhoused animal is best kept in the open, rather than confined to a badly ventilated stable or draughty shed. A blanket may be placed under the rug to provide extra warmth, and the legs can be bandaged with Newmarket bandages. Steam inhalations and mustard plasters or other stimulant applications to the chest are of some value, and the latter will ease discomfort if pleurisy is present. Under no circumstances should the horse be drenched. Soft and nutritious food should be offered in small quantities and varied. Freshly prepared bran mashes, carrots and chopped greenstuff may all be tried in turn. The object is to tempt the horse to eat and so maintain its strength. An adequate and fresh water supply should be readily available.

POISONING
PLANT POISONING

OTHER than Kimberley horse disease and Birdsville disease, which occur in Northern Australia, cases of poisoning of plant origin are far less common in horses than they are in sheep and cattle. Generally, horses are rather selective grazers and are not so prone to eat poisonous plants as are other grazing animals.

Plant poisoning has been discussed at length in my book *Sheep Management and Diseases*, in which is also given a list of the more common poisonous plants in Australia. The subject is also dealt with in my recent book *Cattle Diseases*. There are a great many poisonous plants, shrubs and trees and there is much yet to be learnt regarding their poisonous properties.

The effects produced by eating poisonous plants vary according

157

to the poison they contain. Some plants cause rapid death owing to the toxic action of the poison. Others are highly irritant to the digestive system causing gastro-enteritis followed by death, whilst others again affect the nervous system or cause locomotory disturbance (staggers and incoordination of movement). Other plants cause photosensitization, which has been discussed under *Photosensitization*.

It is frequently difficult, from the symptoms shown by the animal, to differentiate plant poisoning from other common diseases, and the fact that there are poisonous plants in the paddock does not mean that the horse has eaten them. Diarrhoea or scouring, for example, is an indication of gastro-intestinal disorder and, although it may be produced by plants containing irritant poisons, it is also a symptom of bacterial infections and may even be caused by eating indigestible feedstuffs. Plants containing prussic acid or nitrate can cause sudden death, but there are a number of other causes of collapse.

It is necessary, in connection with a suspected case of plant poisoning, to enquire closely into the history of the horse or horses, how hungry they were when turned into a paddock, and to find evidence that they had eaten poisonous plants in sufficient quantity to cause toxicity. If mortality has occurred, a post-mortem examination may help in arriving at a diagnosis.

Stomach contents can be collected and forwarded in a suitable container, preferably a screw-top jar, to a botanist, who may be able to identify the plants which have been eaten. A space should be left at the top to allow for gas formation and a little pure formalin added to reduce fermentation. Specimens of suspected poisonous plants, pressed between newspaper, should also be sent with the stomach contents.

Treatment

The poisonous properties of many plants are not known, which renders treatment difficult. Antidotes are available for only a few kinds of plant poisoning and, to be effective, the diagnosis must be correct and the antidote administered quickly. Professional assistance should be obtained without delay if poisoning is suspected. A drench of $\frac{1}{2}$ lb. of Epsom salts and 4 to 8 oz. of sodium bicarbonate (baking soda) may be of assistance in some plant poisonings. Tannin, in the form of tannic acid ($\frac{1}{2}$ oz.), or strong tea, counteracts many poisons.

See also *Kimberley* or *Walkabout Disease* and *Photosensitization*

MINERAL POISONING

ARSENIC POISONING

Cases of mineral poisoning occur from time to time in horses. Of the mineral poisons, arsenic is the one most commonly responsible for mortality in cattle and sheep in Australia, and has caused deaths of horses. The usual sources of arsenic are sheep and cattle dips from which horses may drink, weed killers, vermin killers, mixtures for painting skins, empty arsenic containers and mining or industrial residues. Pastures that have been poisoned by arsenic from recently dipped sheep and cattle, or vegetation that has been sprayed with arsenical weed killers are sources of poisoning. Horses have suffered from arsenical poisoning from over-dosing with tonic medicines containing arsenic, and also from application of arsenical preparations to the skin.

Symptoms

There are at least four distinct forms of arsenical poisoning, namely *acute, sub-acute, nervous* and *chronic*. In the first category may be included those cases in which death occurs within 36 hours after eating or drinking the arsenic. The symptoms shown are slobbering at the mouth, thirst, loss of appetite, colicky pains, diarrhoea, coldness of the extremities, paralysis of the hindquarters and collapse. Some of these symptoms may not be exhibited and, when a large dose of soluble arsenic has been consumed, the horse may die before the signs of enteritis are shown. In the sub-acute form, the symptoms are somewhat similar but more prolonged; the more prominent are diarrhoea, loss of appetite and disinclination to move. The course of the disease in these cases may extend over two to three days to a week. In the less frequent nervous form of arsenical poisoning, the foregoing symptoms are almost entirely absent. There may be muscular tremor and incoordination, but frequently the animal collapses suddenly without any premonitory symptoms. In such cases, the arsenic appears to paralyse the action of the heart by some direct effect upon the nervous system. The chronic form, sometimes seen in man, is rather rare in stock under Australian conditions. It occurs in other countries where animals are grazed in the vicinity of smelting works and where the water and pasture have become contaminated with arsenic. It can occur, however, where pastures have been contaminated by the drippings from sheep and cattle which have been dipped in an arsenical solution, or on pastures which have been sprayed with an arsenical weed killer. The symptoms shown in this form are poor appetite, intermittent diarrhoea and constipation, wasting, swelling of the joints and loss of hair. There may be reddening of the eyes and swelling of the eyelids and also inflammation and ulceration of the mouth extending sometimes to the muzzle.

Treatment

In the case of acute poisoning, treatment will be of little value unless promptly carried out. Veterinary surgeons have at their disposal a preparation known as *B.A.L.* (British Anti-Lewisite) which, if injected promptly in correct dose rates, has been found a useful antidote for arsenic and some other metallic poisonings. Sodium thiosulphate (photographic hypo), as used for the treatment of arsenical poisoning in sheep and cattle, can also be used for horses. The dose is 1 to 2 oz. given as a drench in $\frac{1}{2}$ a pint of water and repeated at six hourly intervals. A veterinary surgeon would inject intravenously—into a vein—a smaller quantity of this drug, depending on the body weight of the horse, and would be likely to obtain much quicker and more effective results. Any treatment may have to be continued for several days before recovery occurs. A purgative drench of 1 pint of raw linseed oil or a quart of paraffin oil may be given on the first day but not repeated, as over-purging is undesirable.

Two pints of milk or limewater can be given as a drench and repeated in two hours. The whites of 12 eggs may also be given. Good nursing is very important and, provided treatment is commenced early and is carried out by, or under the supervision of a veterinarian, good results can be anticipated, at least in the less acute cases of arsenical poisoning.

LEAD POISONING

This form of poisoning does not occur as frequently in horses as in cattle and, since the advent of new formulations for paints, is not as common in the latter animals as it was. Acute lead poisoning is very rare, but, as lead is a cumulative poison, horses may suffer from the chronic form if they have, over a period, been drinking water that has been standing in new lead pipes, in old lead paint barrels or similar containers. It has occurred when horses have grazed on pastures which have been contaminated by lead residues from smelting works. Horses, unlike cattle, are less liable to lick lead-based painted surfaces, discarded storage batteries, lead foil, pipes and fittings, unless they are suffering from some mineral deficiency. There are cases on record where the source of lead has been from lead arsenate used as a spray in gardens or orchards.

Symptoms

In acute lead poisoning, there are symptoms of abdominal pain, staggering, grinding of the teeth, depression, twitching, especially of the eyelids, champing of the jaws, convulsions and collapse. Chronic lead poisoning leads to loss of appetite, emaciation, constipation and, in some cases, to paralysis of the lower lip and paralysis of part of the larynx, resulting in "roaring".

160

Treatment

The modern treatment for lead poisoning is the use of a complex therapeutic agent sold under the proprietary name of *Calcium Versenate*, which removes absorbed lead from the tissues. The drug is administered in solution by slow intravenous injection over several days and would require the services of a veterinarian. Home remedies consist of a large dose of Epsom salts (10 to 12 oz.) in a pint of water, followed by the administration of milk and whites of eggs in an attempt to prevent further toxic absorption. Oils must not be given. Chronic poisoning may be relieved to some extent by giving 2 to 3 oz. of Epsom or Glauber's salts daily in the drinking water for long periods.

POLL EVIL

See *Fistulous Withers* and *Poll Evil*

POLYPS

THESE are tumours or growths with narrow bases which sometimes occur in cavities like the nose or throat. The name refers to the shape of the growth and has nothing to do with its structure. Most polyps are non-malignant. In the nose, the stem or base of the tumour is generally attached to the membrane high up in the nasal chambers, and when small it cannot be seen. Occasionally it increases in size until it can be observed within the nostril. Sometimes, instead of hanging down towards the nasal opening, it falls back into the pharynx. A polyp may also be attached to the fauces (opening of the back part of the mouth) and the body of the tumour then falls into the pharynx. In this situation, it may seriously interfere with breathing.

Symptoms

When in the nose, these growths cause a peculiar snoring noise, a discharge from the nostril, which may be blood-stained if the tumour is injured, or foetid if the turbinate bones are involved. If the growths are in the throat, the symptoms depend on their location. Interference with breathing is a general symptom, especially if the tumour falls into the pharynx.

Sometimes it falls into the larynx, causing most alarming symptoms. The animal coughs or tries to cough, saliva flows from the mouth, breathing is performed with great difficulty, and accompanied by a loud noise. The animal appears as if strangled and often falls to the ground exhausted. When the tumour is coughed out of the larynx, the animal quickly recovers and soon appears to be quite normal.

161

These sudden attacks and quick recoveries point to the nature of the trouble.

Treatment

These polyps, because of their shape, are comparatively easily removed by a veterinarian.

PREGNANCY

PREGNANCY or gestation is the period during which the female carries its young and when the foetus is undergoing development. The breeding season for horses in Australia starts in September and extends to December or early January. This is because mares normally come into *oestrus* (heat) in the spring and early summer months. At other times the appearance of *oestrus* in mares is irregular, but it can occur at any time of the year. Mares come in season six to nine days after foaling and are commonly mated again at this period. The heat period lasts from three to seven days, but is most variable. In some mares it may be shorter and in others it may last two or three weeks. From the time a mare goes off *oestrus*, a period of sixteen to seventeen days elapses before the next *oestrus* period starts, and, unless the mare is served and gets in foal, this cycle continues throughout the breeding season. The gestation period for mares is about 340 days (329 to 346) or approximately eleven months. This may vary even more, when it is usually associated with some disease of the genital organs.

Indications of Pregnancy

As the mere fact of service by the stallion does not ensure pregnancy, it is important that the result should be determined as soon as possible. A veterinarian can make a fairly accurate diagnosis of pregnancy in a mare by rectal examination, or with greater accuracy by laboratory tests on samples of blood or urine. When this is not done, it is usual to accept the cessation of *oestrus* as evidence of pregnancy, but this is not an infallible sign. Sometimes the mare shows signs of *oestrus* after she has conceived. These symptoms usually only last about a day. Other mares may cease to show signs of *oestrus* and yet have failed to get in foal. An early sign of pregnancy is the altered behaviour of the mare. She usually becomes more docile and tractable after conception and may exhibit other signs, such as change in attitude to other horses. From the third to fourth month onwards, a veterinary surgeon is able to palpate the foetus through the wall of the rectum, but this is not easy in the early stages. Enlargement of the abdomen may be noted at about the fifth month and is more pronounced at six months. Slight falling-in beneath the loins and hollowness of the back are suggestive signs, although they are not always present. Swelling and firmness of the udder, with smoothing out of wrinkles, occur at intervals during gestation. A steady increase in weight, of one to two pounds daily, from about the fifth month is an indication of pregnancy. After the seventh or eighth month, movement of the unborn foal may be detected by pressing firmly with the palm or knuckles of the hand against the abdominal wall in front of the left stifle, especially after the mare has had a drink of water or while she is feeding. The indications of approaching parturition have been described under *Parturition*.

PURPURA HAEMORRHAGICA

THIS is a non-contagious disease which is also known as petechial fever. It may occur following an attack of strangles, influenza or other acute infectious disease. It may also follow upon a deep-seated infected injury, or when a horse is affected with fistulous withers or poll evil. Occasionally it occurs as a primary disease.

The disease damages the walls of the small blood vessels leading to escape of plasma and blood into the tissues. The formation of haemorrhages and the accumulation of dropsical fluid in various parts of the body are characteristic of the condition. It is a serious disease and has a high mortality rate.

Cause

Although the disease has been recognized for a long time, its exact cause is not yet known. Several theories have been advanced. One is that it occurs as the result of a hypersensitive reaction to the protein of streptococcal organisms.

Symptoms

The disease usually appears quite suddenly with, at first, the appearance of small haemorrhages or petechiae on the visible mucous membranes of the nostrils, eyes, mouth and lips of the vulva in mares. This is followed by the development of a dropsical swelling of the nostrils extending over the nose, and sometimes of the eyelids which may later involve the whole head, which then becomes greatly enlarged. The legs swell, and swellings may occur along the belly and on other parts of the body. These swellings tend to disappear quite suddenly and then to reappear later. They are cold and painless and, if pressed with the finger, an indentation remains for a while. On their surface the skin may be tightly stretched and sometimes oozes a pale straw-coloured fluid. Blood may ooze from the haemorrhagic areas and a nasal discharge is quite common. There is variable fever and the horse loses its appetite and becomes weak. The

M

oedematous swellings and haemorrhages may extend internally, leading to pulmonary oedema, or when the intestines are involved, cause a severe attack of colic. Both of these conditions are usually fatal.

The course of an uncomplicated case of the disease is eight to ten days when some cases terminate favourably. In other cases recovery may occur after one or two relapses extending over several weeks. Many horses die well within this period from asphyxia (when oedema of the head is severe), oedema of the viscera, broncho-pneumonia, blood loss, or secondary bacterial infections. The mortality rate is variable, depending on the severity of the cases, but is estimated at approximately fifty per cent.

Treatment

There is evidence to show that the high mortality rate from purpura haemorrhagica is greatly reduced by good treatment and nursing. The treatment therefore requires the co-operation of the veterinary surgeon and the horse-owner. Blood transfusions and heavy antibiotic treatment give the best results. Intravenous injections of calcium gluconate (100 to 200 ml. of a $7 \cdot 5$ per cent solution) daily, have been found useful. No medicine should be given by the mouth owing to the risk of mechanical pneumonia. Good nursing is essential. The horse should be made as comfortable as possible and kept warm, either in the open or in a well-ventilated stable, but the legs should not be bandaged and care is necessary to avoid chafing the swellings with rugs. Clean drinking water should be readily available and kept fresh by frequent changes. To maintain the horse's strength, tempting laxative foods should be fed, such as freshly prepared bran mashes to which scalded oats and sliced carrots may be added. A little green lucerne is useful. If feeding is difficult, owing to swelling of the lips and nose, sloppy foods such as gruels of oatmeal and linseed can be offered. Gentle massage of the swollen limbs, careful grooming with a soft body brush and light exercise are helpful in reducing the oedematous swellings. Care is necessary during the convalescent period to prevent a relapse and a long period of rest is desirable.

QUEENSLAND ITCH

A SKIN disease of horses known as Queensland Itch has been recognized in Australia for a long time, but the cause was not understood and the empirical treatment carried out was not very successful. It was known, however, that when affected horses from the coastal districts of Queensland and New South Wales were sent inland, the disease cleared up. Research work having shown the cause of the disease gives the answer as to why this occurs.

The disease occurs mainly in the summer rainfall areas of the continent, particularly in the coastal and subcoastal regions of Queensland and northern New South Wales, but also elsewhere in coastal or near-coastal regions. It does not occur inland.

Cause

The disease is caused by the hypersensitivity of some horses to the bites of the sandfly, *Culicoides robertsi*. All horses are not affected by the sensitizing substance injected by the sandflies. Susceptible horses, however, show signs of the disease from early summer until the cooler weather approaches. All types, colours and ages of horses are affected by this allergic dermatitis, which is often mistaken for a form of mange.

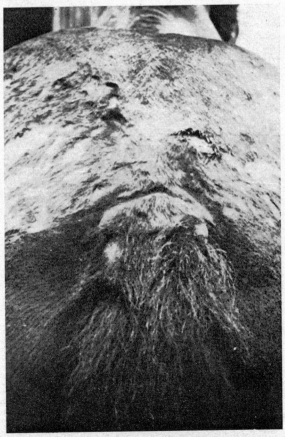

Fig. 68 Queensland Itch. *(Photo Dr. R. F. Riek)*

Symptoms

The lesions are mainly confined to the upper parts of the body including the butt of the tail, rump, along the back, withers, crest, poll and ears. Rarely are lesions found on the sides of the body, the neck, face or legs. Usually the first symptoms shown are the formation of small papules or pimples on which the hair stands erect. The hair on these pimples is brittle and gradually falls out. The itching caused is variable and occurs particularly at night. When severe, the animal rubs the part on any suitable object such as fences and trees and bites at the part if it can reach it, thus aggravating the condition and causing large hairless patches on the body. In chronic cases, the skin becomes thickened and may form into ridges. There is no constitutional disturbance and the appetite is unimpaired, except when secondary bacterial infection of the lesions occurs. Loss of condition may occur as a result of the prolonged irritation and interference with feeding.

Treatment

Frequent intramuscular injections of antihistamines have been shown to relieve the irritation caused by Queensland itch, but would be too costly for general use. The application of antihistamine ointments or creams to the affected areas will relieve the itching and assist cure and subsequent growth of hair.

Prevention of the disease lies in spraying susceptible horses once a week with 1 to 2 per cent solutions of *DDT* dispersible powder in water. The stronger solution is desirable during periods of heavy rain and for horses with short hair, as *DDT* residues are lost more rapidly on short haired animals. A weak solution of *BHC* (1 in 1,000) such as *Gammawash* (I.C.I.) used as a spray once a week, will also protect horses against sandflies. When affected horses are removed to an inland district, the trouble usually clears up.

QUIDDING

WHEN a horse chews its food partially and then drops it from the mouth, it is said to be *quidding*. This generally results from irregular or diseased teeth, or when permanent teeth are pushing the temporary teeth out from the gums. It may also result from abrasions of the membranes of the mouth and tongue or more severe injury to the latter. It can arise from paralysis of the throat or some other condition such as a sore throat, which causes difficulty in swallowing.

Treatment

Quidding is, of course, only a symptom and not a disease. The mouth and throat should be inspected, preferably with a mouth-gag.

166

Dental irregularity must be corrected either by rasping or, if necessary, the extraction of a diseased or projecting tooth (see *Teeth*). Injuries to the mouth and tongue will need attention as will a sore throat. Under certain circumstances, as in the cases of injuries to the mouth, it may be necessary to feed only soft or liquid foods for a few days.

QUITTOR

QUITTOR is the name given to a fistulous wound of the foot opening at the coronet with pus discharging from one or more sinuses.

Causes

The condition results from an infected injury such as a tread on the coronet, a suppurating corn, a punctured wound of the foot and so on. The suppuration usually results initially from a necrotic lateral cartilage.

Symptoms

A quittor causes intense pain and lameness. A greyish coloured pus, often streaked with blood, is discharged almost constantly at the swollen coronet. It is not uncommon, however, for one discharging site at the coronet to heal up, to be followed by pus breaking out at another place. If not checked by efficient treatment, the pus continues to burrow downwards involving other structures.

Treatment

Drainage of pus from the area is the problem in the treatment of quittor. In some early cases, opening up the wound to afford simple drainage, antiseptic treatment and the intramuscular injection of antibiotics may bring about favourable results. Repeated hot fomentations and poulticing may be applied to advantage in certain cases.

Most cases of quittor need expert surgery under an anaesthetic to remove all diseased tissue, including sometimes the whole of the lateral cartilage. Frequent dressing of the surgical wound is then necessary and the convalescent period may be quite prolonged. Cartilage is poorly nourished by blood and once it is injured and infected, necrosis or death of the part commonly occurs, hence the difficulty of bringing about a cure without surgery. Healing cannot take place until the area or areas either slough away or are surgically removed.

RETENTION OF AFTERBIRTH

THE AFTERBIRTH or "cleansing" refers to the foetal membranes (placenta) in which the foetus develops in the uterus (womb), which serve as a connection between it and the mother. It is composed of three parts, the *chorion*, the *amnion* and the *allantois*, which are expelled when, or soon after, the young animal is born. The term placenta refers to the special area of the membranes through which the blood circulation of the mother nourishes the foetus.

Retention of the afterbirth in the mare is much less frequent, but much more serious than in the cow. In the mare the afterbirth is normally expelled regularly a few hours after the foal is born, but if the mare has not "cleaned" properly within six to eight hours, action must be taken to remove the membranes manually, otherwise infection is likely to occur. Owing to the speed with which the membranes decompose, and the risk of death of the mare or the development of metritis and acute laminitis, a veterinarian should be called immediately. If a veterinarian is not available and the horse-owner is obliged to attempt to remove the membranes, the greatest cleanliness and antiseptic precautions must be taken.

If portion of the membranes are protruding, it may be possible to remove them without introducing the hand into the uterus, thus avoiding introduction of infection. Examine the part hanging out and separate the more bulky, comparatively thin, and whitish-grey portion from the lesser, thicker and reddish-coloured portion. Collect within the hand as much of the reddish and thicker portion as possible. Wrap this around the thinner greyish membranes so that the free portion of the reddish membrane, now outermost, represents the layer previously adherent to the wall of the uterus. Now commence to twist the afterbirth, keeping the reddish portion outermost, and at the same time exerting gentle traction to keep the membranes moving steadily through the vulva. This torsion is continued slowly until all the afterbirth has been removed. If this is done hurriedly, haemorrhage is likely to occur. In order to be sure that the whole of the afterbirth has been removed, spread the membranes out and find the opening of the sac at the end which first protruded. Now pour a gallon of water into this opening and lift up the membranes sufficiently high to let the water run into the two uterine horns. These should be intact so that the afterbirth holds water and appears something like a pair of trousers tied at the ends of the legs. If any portion is missing it will be necessary to pass the thoroughly-cleaned hand (with short-cut fingernails) and arm into the uterus and horns in order to gently remove the retained portions.

Douching out the uterus with weak antiseptic solution is not now advocated.

The best method of controlling infection is the insertion of soluble, wide-spectrum antibiotic pessaries into the uterus, combined with antibiotics administered intramuscularly.

RETENTION OF URINE

See *Suppression of Urine*

RIG

A RIG is a horse in which one or both testicles have failed to come down into the scrotum. In the foal, the descent of the testicles is often complete at birth, but it frequently happens that one testicle or both may be retained for months in the inguinal canal or in the abdomen. In other cases the testicle may descend normally but return into the canal or abdomen. This may occur because the ring through which the testicle passes is large, and the testicle small and soft and not yet closely anchored down by the scrotal ligament. It is for this reason that colts are not castrated until they are twelve months old or more. Indefinite retention of one testicle or both is not uncommon. This condition is termed cryptorchidism and the animal is commonly referred to as a "rig".

A testicle which is retained in the inguinal canal or the abdomen does not produce fertile spermatozoa because of the body temperature to which it is exposed.

If only one testicle is retained, the stallion may still be fertile, but if both are retained, he will be sterile. A cryptorchid horse is a nuisance and is often difficult to handle. The male hormone, *testosterone*, has been used for correction of retained testicles. However, if the retained testicle has not descended by the time the colt is two years old, a cryptorchid operation by a veterinary surgeon will be necessary. This is best done when the colt is rising three years old.

RINGBONE

RINGBONE is an exostosis (bony outgrowth) just above the top of the hoof, affecting the joint between the pedal bone and the short pastern bone. The bony enlargement may extend around the joint, hence the name. This is sometimes referred to as low ringbone. Similar bony outgrowths occur on the long pastern bone or the joint between the long and short pastern bones. This is commonly termed high ringbone. Low ringbone must not be confused with sidebone, which is a hardening of the lateral cartilages of the foot and is dealt with under *Sidebones*. Ringbone is more common on the fore feet than on the hind feet.

Cause

Heredity plays an important part in the cause of ringbone, and the conformation of the legs induces liability to the disease. Other possible

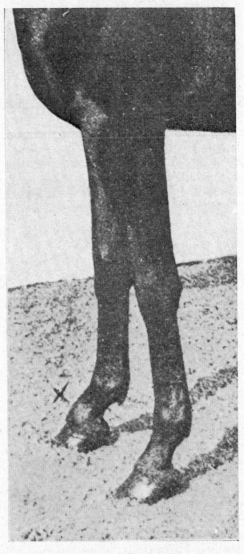

Fig. 69   Ringbone at X.

(*United States Department of Agriculture*)

causes are heavy working of a young horse before the process of ossification has fully occurred; bruises; blows; sprains or injuries of tendons, ligaments and joints. All the latter are secondary to heredity and conformation.

Symptoms

Lameness, which may occur before there are any obvious signs of the trouble. The lameness of ringbone is especially manifested when the affected animal is required to step from side to side. Marked flinching then occurs when weight is borne on the affected leg, even though no lameness may be revealed when the animal goes in a straight line. The lameness is frequently irregular at first, but finally becomes more or less constant and is accompanied by a plainly-visible, bony enlargement of the pastern. In the early stages of low ringbone, there may be heat and pain at the hoof-head, and bending of the joint causes increase of pain.

Treatment

The treatment of ringbone is generally unsatisfactory. Firing and blistering in the early stages may arrest the condition and cause the absorption of the bony material which has already been deposited. A long rest on soft ground is essential after this treatment. The usual outcome of the disease is the formation of sufficient bony material to cause ankylosis, or complete fusion of the bones of a part or all of the involved joint, thus destroying the free action of the affected joint. In such cases, serviceability rather than complete cure is aimed at. Specially-designed shoes can be fitted for such cases, in conjunction with changing of the proportions or angles of the hoof by appropriate trimming. Neurotomy—cutting out a piece of nerve—may be carried out to prolong the usefulness of the horse for a short time, if considered justifiable.

RINGWORM

RINGWORM is a contagious skin disease brought about by the growth of fungi on the skin and at the roots of hairs, and may be caused by a number of species. The disease is spread by direct contact with infected animals or contaminated objects such as bedding, harness and saddles, grooming kits, horse blankets, rails and fences. It can be a very troublesome disease when large numbers of horses are brought together as occurred during the two World Wars. Fungal spores are very resistant and may survive in stalls and sheds for a year or longer. Spores can also exist on the skin of animals without causing the disease, so that apparently-healthy animals can act as carriers. Minor abrasions of the skin surface may favour infection.

The incubation period after a natural infection is generally from a week to a month. Ringworm is readily transmissible from animals to man.

Symptoms

When the hairs and their roots are invaded by the fungus of ringworm, the hairs break off short. Small bare areas are then formed which later spread from the outer boundary, thus giving the area its characteristic circular appearance from which the name is derived. Not infrequently, the small bald spots which occur in the early stages of ringworm, on almost any part of the body of the horse, are apt to be regarded as of no consequence and due to minor injuries. The subsequent appearance of the lesions varies somewhat according to the species of fungi. The skin of the bare area may become raised and scurfy, and greyish-white crusts form, giving the area a scaly appearance. The area heals in the centre, but fresh areas occur around the outside edge. Itching is not great, although the horse may show some signs of irritation by rubbing against objects. In another type of ringworm, pustules are formed below the crusts and the itchiness is much greater. It is not uncommon for ringworm lesions to join up and form large irregular-shaped bare areas over the head and body.

A definite diagnosis of ringworm can be readily made from examination of skin scrapings under a microscope.

Treatment

Because ringworm is a self-limiting disease and spontaneous recovery is likely to occur over a period, doubt has been expressed as to the value of any treatment for ringworm. Nevertheless, treatment, if well carried out, will arrest the spread of the disease and

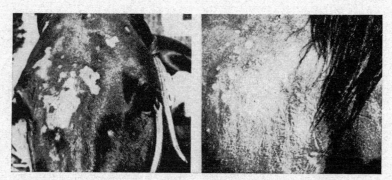

Fig. 70 Ringworm.
(From Equine Medicine and Surgery, American Veterinary Publications Inc.)

172

this can be important. There are many preparations on the market for the topical treatment of ringworm and most of them have to be well scrubbed in with a hard-bristled brush. Where the disease is detected early and there are only a few lesions, the hair over and around the part should be clipped and the clippings collected and burnt. Now soften the scaly crusts with warm soapy water, or two ounces of washing soda to a pint of water, followed by scraping or brushing. After drying, one of the effective fungicidal preparations should be brushed or well rubbed into the lesions, paying particular attention to the outside edges. Tincture of iodine well brushed in every other day has been found to be effective in some cases, but not in others. Whitfields Ointment, or ten per cent ammoniated mercury ointment, and many other dressings are used, but none has been shown to be outstanding. There are a number of new anti-fungal agents on the market which are said to be effective in the treatment of ringworm, but which should preferably be used under veterinary supervision. Griseofulvin, a new antibiotic with powerful anti-fungal properties, has been found to be an effective though rather expensive form of treatment. It is available in tablet form for administration by the mouth under various proprietary names such as *Grisovin*, *Fulcin* and *Fulcinfort*. A new preparation, *Camdogon,* is now available, which is said not to require softening of the scabs and which may be sprayed onto the lesions or applied with a soft brush.

When infection is widespread in a large number of horses, as occurred in the Army during the Second World War, the only practical way of dealing with the problem is to apply washes or sprays over the entire body surface of all animals in an attempt to treat, or at least control the spread of infection. Agricultural Bordeaux mixture was used on the army horses, being prepared as follows:

   2 lb. of copper sulphate (bluestone) dissolved in 20 gallons
       of water

   2 lb. of fresh unslaked hydrated lime mixed in 20 gallons of
       water

The two mixtures were then mixed in a wooden vat and stirred until a test with litmus paper indicated an alkaline reaction. Spraying with a hand spray at five-day intervals was recommended. Although the results were not entirely satisfactory, the disease was checked, and in some groups after only two treatments. A good deal depends on the thoroughness with which the spray is applied. Where practicable, it is desirable to scrub the mixture into the lesions with a stiff brush.

Owing to the possibility of transmission of the disease to man, the hands and arms should be thoroughly washed after attending cases of ringworm.

Control

In addition to the measures outlined under "treatment", affected horses should be treated as soon as they are found and segregated until the lesions have healed. The premises of stabled horses and all grooming equipment, harness, saddles and rugs should be cleaned and disinfected.

ROARING AND WHISTLING

THESE are chronic conditions which are characterized by an unnatural noise that can be heard when the horse is breathing deeply from exertion. The only difference is the pitch of the note, which is higher in whistling than in roaring. The noise is made during inspiration of air into the lungs and in severe cases may be accompanied by difficult or laboured breathing. The condition is seen most commonly in thoroughbred and other light horses. It is rare in ponies and mules. The incidence is greatest in animals three to six years old.

Cause

Whereas heredity plays an important part as a predisposing cause of roaring, especially in long-necked horses, it may be an acquired characteristic brought on following an attack of strangles, laryngitis, bronchitis and so on. It may also result from lead poisoning.

The immediate cause is degeneration of one or both of the recurrent laryngeal nerves giving rise to partial or complete paralysis of the muscles of the larynx, usually on the left side. Temporary roaring can occur due to inflammation and thickening of the mucous lining of the larynx caused by various respiratory diseases. This is not to be confused with the chronic condition.

Symptoms

In chronic roaring there is no sign of any disease of the larynx, although an experienced veterinarian may, by palpation, be able to detect evidence of the wasted condition of the muscles in question. Unless the muscles on both sides of the larynx are affected, the horse shows no symptoms when at rest, but if a light horse is galloped some distance, or a draught horse made to pull a heavy load uphill, the roaring or whistling sound on inspiration is soon evident. Whistling is not as serious a condition as roaring and, under stress, a roarer shows symptoms earlier than a whistler. A horse that whistles may

174

develop into a roarer. In the early stages of the disease, and before symptoms of whistling or roaring are shown, some horses give a characteristic grunt when frightened or when struck a sudden blow over the ribs.

Treatment

There is no medicinal treatment for chronic roaring or whistling, as it is impossible to restore the degenerated nerve or the wasted muscle. Various operations are carried out to overcome the roaring, including stripping the lining membrane from a little pouch which lies between the vocal cord and the laryngeal wall, with the object of encouraging the vocal fold to adhere to the wall of the larynx out of the path of the entering stream of air.

As an alternative, the operation of tracheotomy can be performed. This consists of cutting out two rings of the windpipe in front and inserting a special tube. With such a tube, a horse can be made serviceable for many years, either for fast or slow work. Horses have even raced successfully with a tube in the windpipe.

RUPTURE

See *Hernia*

SADDLE GALLS—SORE BACKS

BECAUSE saddle galls are so common in riding horses and there is lack of understanding am~~ong owners in p~~articular, of the cause of these galls or sores on the back, the subject is dealt with at length.

Cause

Saddle galls are caused by friction or pressure due to a badly-fitting saddle. They are associated very often with wasting of the back muscles when the horse falls away in condition, or conversely when the horse puts on condition, is fat and soft, and sweats easily when worked. A horse properly fed and in hard-working condition can stand much more friction and pressure than one in soft condition. Bad riding may be a cause. Unaccustomed and prolonged pressure causes chafing or a break in the skin, thus paving the way for infection. Chafing, if long continued, may lead to a callosity. This may be superficial, involving only the skin, or it may be deep-seated and cause a sitfast.

To fully appreciate why saddles so often cause injuries, it is necessary to have some knowledge of the parts where the injuries occur, and where pressure and weight can be applied with the minimum likelihood of injury. A very useful little book published many years ago by the Veterinary Department of the War Office, London, called *Animal Management* and used in the Australian Army Veterinary Corps, contains much useful information on the subject of saddles and sore backs. Much of the following discussion on the anatomical construction of the back in relation to saddle fitting is based on this book, with due acknowledgement, bearing in mind the use of an ordinary riding saddle.

Structure of the Back

The spine is composed of a chain of bones which have limited movement. The movements of the spinal chain are upwards and downwards and from side to side. This is illustrated when a horse bucks and his spine arches, or when the spine becomes depressed under the influence of weight. It moves from side to side when an animal turns to the right or left, especially in flag races, polo and other games. The bones of the back comprise eighteen links closely knitted together. The spine is distinctly arched, rising from the neck bones and falling again towards the hindquarters. This arched arrangement provides strength, but actually the spine of man, which is vertical, is much more capable of carrying weight than the horizontal spine of the horse.

The back and loins are frequently confused in the minds of some people, and it is necessary when considering the matter of carrying weight that novices in particular should be differentiated. The back bones extend from the last bone of the neck to the last rib. The loins lie between the last rib and the quarters. A great deal of the backbone is out of sight, being covered by the shoulders or blade-bones. The portion of back which is visible extends from the play of the blade-bones to the last rib, and this is the part which is of so much interest in saddle fitting.

Throughout the whole length of the spine, vertical bony processes occur, which grow from the upper part of each vertebra or link of the chain. The processes in front are very long and their summits form the withers. Those behind are short and broad. The front processes project backward, those behind project forward. The tops of the bony processes form the ridge of the backbone. They do not represent the spine proper, the links of which are more deeply seated, but they are the only part which can be felt, and are the site of bone trouble which may follow a bad sore back. An important point to keep in mind is that these bony processes should not bear weight.

176

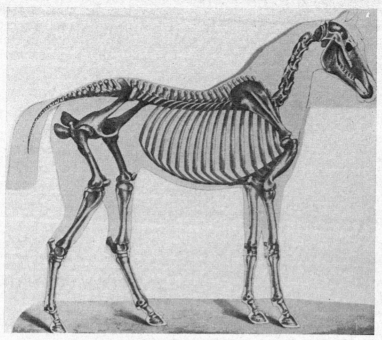

Fig. 71 The Skeleton of the Horse.

(*After Schwarz and Fleming*)

The Ribs

These are attached to the backbone by joints, thus allowing the ribs to move. They are eighteen in number and are divided into eight true ribs and ten so-called "false ribs". The true ribs extend directly to the sternum (breastbone) by the rib cartilages. The remaining ten ribs do not extend to the breastbone at all and for this reason are called "false ribs". The true ribs are stout and nearly straight, the false ribs are thinner and curved. The curving and arching of the ribs increases from front to rear so that the chest is narrowest between the front two ribs and widest between the last two. A true rib is stronger than a false one and has much less movement.

In saddle fitting advantage is taken of the true ribs being fitted into the breastbone. The ribs move with each act of breathing, the movement, broadly, being forwards and backwards. The ribs in front move very little, those behind move freely. *When a saddle is placed on the back, it rests on the ribs, and it is on the ribs and not on the spine that the weight is actually carried.* This fundamental fact is the basis of all saddle fitting. The rear ribs carry the weight on their upper surface, but the front ribs, being stouter and fixed into the

177

breastbone, can carry weight not only on their upper surface, but also on their side. If it were not for these ribs being fixed into the breastbone, a girth could not be used.

The Loins

The bones of the loins are usually six in number (sometimes five) and in several respects resemble the links of the backbone. They are larger and have, growing out from them horizontally on each side, a thin, flat plate of bone, but there are no ribs. On the length of these bony plates, known as the transverse processes, depends the width of the loins. *The loins are not suitably constructed to support weight, and no weight should ever rest on them.* They do, however, have a function to perform in connection with weight carrying, which will be referred to later.

The Forelegs

The forelegs of the horse are not joined to the body by means of a joint, but are attached to the trunk by means of large masses of muscle. The trunk of the horse is therefore slung between the forelegs and in this respect they differ from the hind legs which are secured to the body by muscles and a large cup-and-ball joint. The muscles which hold the forelegs to the body are spread over the sides of the ribs to which they are firmly attached. The upper bone of the foreleg, the scapula or so-called blade-bone, is shaped something like a fan and lies flat on the surface of the ribs. When the foreleg moves, the blade-bone moves, its range of movement being greater near the shoulder-joint than above. The movement of the blade-bone is forwards and backwards. Bearing the above points in mind, it will be apparent that, as the blade-bone is travelling to and fro, nothing which is placed on a horse's back in the form of a saddle should ever press upon it or interfere with its movements, otherwise the length and safety of the horse's stride will be affected.

Back Muscles

A large slab of muscles runs the whole length of the back and loins, filling up the triangular space between the processes of the vertebrae and the ribs. It is on this slab of muscles that the saddle rests and, from a saddle-fitting point of view, it is most important. Beneath the skin is a thin, tough, yellow elastic layer of material, which spreads like a sheet over the loins and back and envelops the muscles, which it hides from view. It is there for the purpose of additional strength, but it is this layer of material which contributes so largely to the difficulties of treating severe sore backs. Infection penetrating beneath the skin from a sore on the back may spread in all directions over this elastic layer. This, coupled with the fact that

178

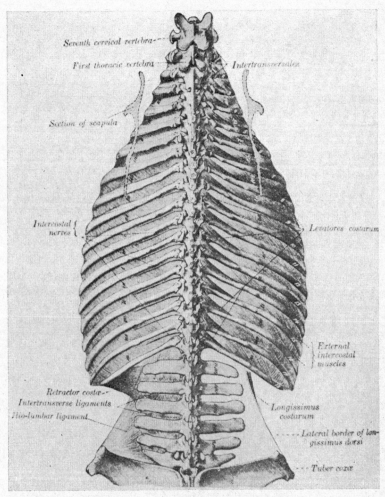

Fig. 72   Deep Dissection of Dorsal and Lumbar Regions of Horse.

(After Schmaltz, Atlas d. Anat. d. Pferdes in Sisson-Grossman,
Anatomy of the Domestic Animals, 4th edition.
Philadelphia, W. B. Saunders Co. 1953)

179

N

there is poor drainage from a wound on the back, means that infected injuries to the back naturally tend to get worse rather than better. It will therefore be seen that, from the anatomical arrangement of the part, wounds of the back are usually slow healing and require treatment for a protracted period.

The Skin

Briefly, there are two layers of skin, an outer composed of scales possessing very little sensation and no blood, and an inner which is highly sensitive and rich in blood vessels. Owing to the hair and colour of the skin, the blood can rarely be seen in a horse's skin as it can in man. The capillary blood vessels are very small and numerous. Their structure is so delicate that very little pressure is necessary to empty the minute blood vessels of blood, as can be well demonstrated by pressure on one's hand with a finger. The influence of this in relation to sore backs will be referred to later.

Shape of the Back

The shape of the back depends entirely on the shape of the bones which compose it. The curve of the spine is represented by the bony processes already described. When these are short, the back tends towards flatness, as in the donkey; when they are long, the withers are high and the ridge of the backbone prominent. These bony processes also determine the slope of the withers—long processes mean high withers, short processes mean thick, low withers. The slope of the back greatly influences the production of injury, and nowhere is it better seen than in the case of the withers. Horses with high withers do not make good saddle horses, and the opposite extreme of low withers is also undesirable, although not quite so objectionable. Long backs are a source of weakness, and as a rule they are poorly developed. These backs are frequently associated with a long narrow loin which is a serious fault if a horse is to carry a person for any length of time. A short back is a sign of strength and is associated with a short, wide loin. Provided the back is long enough for the saddle, it can be said that the loin can hardly be too short. High withers are generally associated with good action, but when excessively high it is not uncommon to find the back hollow. Furthermore, high withers are always lean and narrow and a horse that has them is always in danger of injury. Low withers may be associated with slow, clumsy action. When the withers are very low, they are also very wide. A wide wither is nearly as troublesome as a high one, not for the reason that it gets pressed upon, as in the case of the high wither, but because it is liable to be pinched. A hollow back is bad for a riding horse, because, owing to the curve, the saddle is unable to get a level bed on the back, with the result that injury follows. A roach back is the converse of a hollow one, and is always a sign of strength, but is most uncomfortable for the rider, and may also be injured by unequal pressures. Wide backs accompany well-arched ribs and afford a good wide bed for the saddle to rest on—an essential formation for a good stock horse. Excessive width must, however, be avoided, as the saddle will work forward on to the neck. Narrow backs are due to poorly-sprung ribs. These ribs are too straight, and in consequence there is very little bearing surface for the saddle. A flat-sided horse, besides carrying his saddle badly, is usually deficient in stamina and soon succumbs to fatigue.

Back Muscles in Relation to the Saddle

A saddle should not directly rest on any of the hard structures of the back, be it spine or ribs. It must rest only on those parts well clothed with muscle, and the only part of the back so clothed is the angular space formed by the ribs and the processes of the vertebrae. In saddle fitting, the muscles of the back act as a buffer to the bones beneath, and so prevent injury. The saddle should not be allowed to rest on any part of the back that has no muscle to protect it, other-

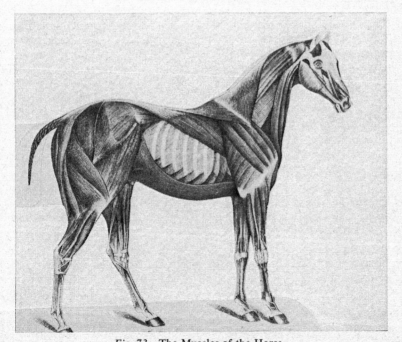

Fig. 73   The Muscles of the Horse.

(*After Schwarz and Fleming*)

181

wise injury results. Back muscles, of course, vary according to the condition of the horse. In a well-nourished and well-cared-for horse, the muscles are large and well developed and afford the maximum of protection. Where the muscles are impoverished and weak due to malnutrition or over-work, saddle injury is likely to occur.

Skin Pressure

Brief reference has already been made to the blood vessels in the skin and how readily pressure acts in keeping these vessels empty. The continuous circulation of blood in the skin ensures the rapid renewal of the skin which, being exposed to friction, would soon wear away to the more sensitive parts unless constantly replaced. There are other functions which the blood and the skin perform, but they are not relevant to this subject. If the blood supply to any part of the body be cut off, the part dies. Whether it dies rapidly or slowly depends on the thoroughness with which the blood supply has been cut off. If complete, the death of the part will take only a few hours; if incomplete it may take a few days. This statement holds good whether it be a limb or a small piece of skin on the back. Pressure will kill any of the tissues of the body.

The skin of the horse's back is subject to pressure when a person mounts, and, in consequence, less blood circulates through it than before. The greater the weight imposed, the greater is the pressure on the skin and, with every increase in pressure, less blood circulates through it. The pressure is not quite the same at any two points over the back. It is greater here and less there, depending upon the fit of the saddle, so that we never expect to see the whole length of the skin on the back die as a result of pressure, but only where the saddletree has been particularly ill-fitting and the pressure the greatest. So long as there is a good deep muscle bed beneath the skin, the chances of completely cutting off the blood supply are very small. If, however, the horse falls away in condition and the back muscles become reduced in bulk, the saddle is brought nearer to the skeleton and the firm, now ill-fitting saddle on the one hand and rigid bone on the other will cause pressures resulting in destruction of the skin.

On the other hand, even if the horse is well muscled and the saddle fits perfectly, injury to the back will result from continuous pressure if the horse is ridden hour after hour and not given relief from its burden.

Saddles

It is impossible to consider saddle injuries and galls without a brief discussion of the saddle generally. A few points only will be dealt with. The framework of a saddle consists of two arches, one in

182

front and one behind the rider. Each arch rests upon and is secured to two bars placed parallel to each other, through the medium of which the rider's weight is distributed on the back of the horse. Two arches are used to ensure that the spine is not pressed upon, and two bars are used by which the arches are kept in their place. The arches are made of wood or metal or a combination of these. The front arch forms the pommel, the rear arch the cantle. Both pommel and cantle may be high or low depending on the type of saddle. The side bars are that portion of the saddle which rests on the back, and to which the front and rear arches are secured. Side bars are generally made of wood, and in military saddles are given a twist in the making which enables them to be adjusted to the curves of the back. The function of a side bar is to afford a firm support for the arches of the saddle and to distribute the weight over the back. Bearing in mind the weight-bearing region, namely from the play of the shoulder to the last rib, it is clear that over this surface the side bars should rest evenly, squarely and without undue pressure at any one point. In the manufacture of the common type of riding saddle, little attention is paid to the curves of the side bar, and the fit of the saddle and distribution of weight are more or less assured by the shape of a panel stuffed with horse-hair and flock.

So far the framework of the saddle has been briefly considered. If this has been constructed to comply with the basic requirements described, and is of sufficient strength to provide a firm foundation, the other parts of the saddle, such as the seat, flaps, panels, *etc.*, become mere accessories.

A sling of webbing between the arches supports the leather of the seat and takes the weight of the rider. The seat is not normally associated with sore backs. It may, however, be a source of injury to the horse if, through the leatherwork stretching or stitches giving way, it comes down on the spine. This may also occur if a horse falls away in condition, allowing the saddle to settle. A tight overgirth is another common cause of seats sinking.

Flaps to a saddle are a convenience but are not absolutely necessary—a blanket would do as well. The saddle flap is rarely a cause of injury. The panels of a plain saddle each consist of a bag made of leather and serge, stuffed with horsehair and flock. In the course of time, they become moulded to the horse's back and adjust themselves to the various irregularities. Well-moulded saddles, if properly looked after, play a part in the prevention of sore backs, but they can cause trouble if they are too bulky or too thin, or if the stuffing has become consolidated, lumpy, or even hardened by accumulation of sweat.

Saddle Blanket

A blanket beneath the saddle is an admirable method of protecting the back. It cannot be used to produce the full effect of graduated variations in thickness achieved by shaped panels, but considerable changes can be brought about by altering the method of folding. A good quality blanket, which folds well and does not wrinkle, should be used. Useful adjustments can be made by altering the folding of a blanket, when back muscles are starting to waste due to the horse falling away in condition, or if the back is injured. A saddle blanket should be used as padding to compensate for any loss of condition, so that the saddle will not settle on to the spine, and to protect the ribs from bruising.

Saddling Faults

The Army book *Animal Management* lays down six axioms in saddle fitting, namely,

"1. The withers must not be pinched or pressed upon.
2. The central line of the back must have no pressure imposed upon it.
3. The blade bones must have free and uncontrolled movement.
4. The loins are not intended to carry weight.
5. The weight must be imposed on the ribs through the medium of the muscles covering them.
6. The weight must be evenly distributed over a surface which extends from the play of the shoulders to the last rib."

It is common to blame a rider for giving a horse a sore back, when actually the fault lies with the saddle or the condition of the horse. Sometimes the fault does lie with the rider, but this is not as common as supposed. Bad saddling is frequently the cause of sore backs, but there is a marked distinction between bad saddling and defective saddle fitting, which has previously been discussed. Under the term "bad saddling" may be included—the blanket or saddle cloth being not properly folded and raised off the backbone—the loose end of any strap getting between the saddle cloth and the skin —the edge of the girth or panel flap being turned in when putting the saddle on in a hurry—a loose girth or a tight surcingle.

General

From the foregoing discussion on sore backs in horses, it will be appreciated that almost every injury to the back is due to either friction or pressure. These act either by wearing away the part by rubbing, by bruising, or by partly or entirely cutting off the blood supply. The condition of the horse greatly influences the production of sore backs. A horse well fed and in hard working condition can stand much more friction and pressure than one in soft condition. The important point is that in nearly every case of injury the cause can be determined and corrected. One hears of certain ointments or lotions that are good for sore backs. That is not important. The main thing is to ascertain the cause and remove it, when in many early cases the horse may be able to continue in work.

A simple gall or erosion of the skin may be cleansed with a weak antiseptic solution, such as *Dettol* or *Cetavlon* and then dabbed repeatedly with an astringent antiseptic lotion, such as white lotion (zinc sulphate 1 oz., lead acetate 1 oz., water 1 pint) which should be well shaken. Mild antiseptic dusting powders may also be used. Frequent bathing is undesirable. When the injury has progressed to a sitfast (chronic, crusted ulcer due to necrosis of the skin), surgical removal of the dead tissue may be necessary. If the bone below is involved, this calls for more extensive surgery.

Where a horse has to be worked with a sore back, chambering of the saddle can be carried out to accommodate the sore. A chamber is a depression made in the panel to take all bearing off the injured place. It must be made accurately, as a chamber badly placed is useless. It is best done by a saddler. Nothing should be placed between the back and the chamber, otherwise the injury will be aggravated.

SALIVARY CALCULI (Cheek Stones)

A CALCULUS ("stone") is sometimes formed in the duct of the parotid salivary gland (*Stenson's duct*), along the side of the face of the horse. It appears as a hard, sharply defined, slightly movable swelling and may attain considerable size. The salivary duct is usually distended behind the swelling and, when the flow of saliva is entirely shut off, the gland beneath the ear becomes enlarged. Inflammation is seldom present, but infection may occur and lead to abscess formation.

Treatment

A minor operation is necessary to remove the calculus, but this should be carried out by a veterinarian.

SANDCRACK

A SANDCRACK is a fissure in the horn of the wall of the foot which commences immediately below the coronary band and extends part of the way or right down the wall. These fissures are narrow and, as a general rule, they follow the direction of the horn fibres. They may occur on any part of the wall, but the common situations are directly in front of the hoof, when they are termed toe cracks, or to the side of the hoof, when they are known as quarter cracks. True toe cracks are most common in the hind feet, whereas quarter cracks nearly always affect the fore feet, where they are seen more commonly on the inside quarter of the foot. The term *complete sandcrack* means that the crack extends from the coronary band to the ground surface. This occurs more commonly in a toe crack than in a quarter crack, which is generally incomplete. The seriousness of sandcracks depends on whether they are superficial, involving only the outer parts of the wall, or whether they are deep, involving the whole thickness of the wall and penetrating to the soft tissues beneath.

Cause

Faulty conformation predisposes a horse to sandcrack, but any horse having dry, brittle hooves is liable to develop the trouble. Furthermore, anything that interferes with the proper secretion of horn at the coronet, such as an injury sustained from a tread, from over-reaching or other accidental wounding of the coronary band, can lead to the condition. Overgrown toes of the hind feet may lead to continual pressure on the coronary substance by the small pastern bone, thus interfering with its function and causing sandcrack. Excessive rasping of the outer surface of the hoof, which renders the horn brittle; alternate changes from damp to dry conditions of standing; excessive dryness and unskilful shoeing, are some of the other predisposing causes. Concussion from fast work on hard roads and jumping, especially in association with other factors, plays a part in the causation of sandcracks and more particularly quarter cracks.

Symptoms

The presence of the crack in the horn is the most obvious symptom. When the crack is superficial, lameness is not shown, but when it is deep, pinching of the soft structures may occur, or infection supervene, causing lameness. Extensive injury to the coronet immediately above the sandcrack causes swelling, which may ultimately give rise to the condition known as false quarter. Various complications can occur following infection of a deep sandcrack.

Treatment

Sandcracks are treated according to their location and extent. In a simple case, where the crack is superficial and close under the coronary margin, blistering of the coronet will stimulate horn growth sufficiently to overcome the crack. Alternatively, the coronet may be clipped immediately above the crack and a horizontal line made one inch long and about a quarter of an inch deep with a hot iron just

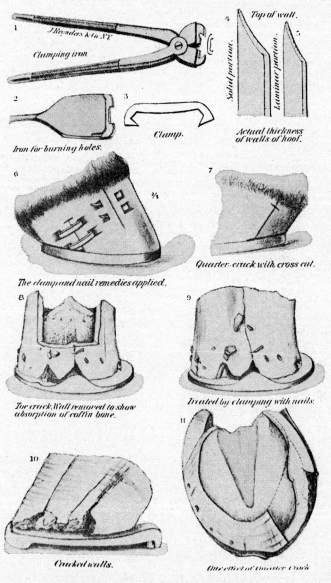

1 J.Reynders & Co. N.Y.

Clamping iron.

2 Iron for burning holes.

3 Clamp.

4 Top of wall.
Solid portion.
Laminar portion.
5
Actual thickness of walls of hoof.

6 ⅔
The clamp and nail remedies applied.

7 Quarter-crack with cross cut.

8 Toe crack.Wall removed to show absorption of coffin bone.

9 Treated by clamping with nails.

10 Cracked walls.

11 One effect of Quarter-Crack.

Fig. 74   Sandcracks and Treatment.

(*From Diseases of the Horse,
United States Department of Agriculture*)

below the coronary band through the upper end of the crack. Afterwards a blister should be applied to the coronary band above the sandcrack. This blister might be repeated to advantage in a fortnight. Before shoeing, the ground surface of the foot where the crack would normally end should be cut away to relieve pressure. For more extensive and wider cracks, special clips may be used to hold the margins of the crack together. A good farrier may accomplish the same thing with well-placed horseshoe nails. Special shoeing is sometimes employed to minimize the effects and even eventually to cure sandcracks. Grooves may be cut around the crack to immobilize the hoof wall, thus permitting healing.

In complicated cases, where infection has occurred and there is acute lameness, hot antiseptic footbaths, or the application of poultices are indicated to reduce the inflammation and help to control the infection. Antibiotics are used to greater advantage in infected cases, and for this reason these cases should receive veterinary attention. If the crack is very complicated and has refused to yield to other forms of treatment, a surgical operation can be carried out under an anaesthetic, when a portion of the horn involved in the crack is removed. A long spell is necessary until new horn fills the uncovered space. Acrylics, a form of "plastic", are now being used to repair injuries and defects in horses' hooves.

SCIRRHOUS CORD

THIS IS a hard fibrous enlargement of the cut end of the spermatic cord in castrated horses.

Cause

The condition is caused by infection of the stump of the spermatic cord by *Staphylococcal* organisms, mainly *Staphylococcus aureus*, at the time of, or shortly after, castration. Chronic abscesses with thick fibrous walls are produced, interspersed with a mass of granulomatous tissue, the whole of which may weigh seven to eight pounds.

Symptoms

The first symptom is usually incomplete healing of the castration wound, some swelling in the region, and the discharge of thick pus. This discharge may cease after a while, but the swelling continues to increase slowly in size. The swelling causes a stiff, straddling gait, and may be felt as a hard mass in the groin, connected above with the cord. It continues to grow slowly for many years, and it is not uncommon for a horse, castrated as a yearling, not to show marked signs of the condition until he is four or five years old.

Treatment

The treatment is surgery under an anaesthetic. Arrangements should be made for the operation to be carried out before the mass has become too large, otherwise it may be impracticable, or cause systemic complications.

SEEDY-TOE

SEEDY-TOE is a condition of the hoof in which there is a separation between the inner and outer parts of the wall, usually at the toe, but occurring elsewhere round the foot. It is a defect in the horn of the wall. The space is partly filled with degenerated crumbly horn, and the cavity may not be seen until the foot is pared after removal of the shoe.

Cause

There has been much speculation as to the cause of seedy-toe, but basically it would appear to be associated with some abnormality of the coronary band following an injury, and interference with the horn-secreting substance. Bacteria and fungi, which have been reported as causing the condition, would appear to be secondary invaders.

Symptoms

Seedy-toe does not usually cause lameness. This does occur, however, when the separation is large and dirt and small stones have become wedged into the space and thus cause pressure on the sensitive laminae. The cavity may be detected in the shod horse by tapping the foot on the outside with a light hammer. Once the cavity is exposed by paring the foot, the extent of the separation can be ascertained with the blade of a pocket knife or a thin nail.

Treatment

A small cavity can be cleaned out, packed with cotton wool and tar and the foot shod in such a way as to relieve pressure over the area. The usual treatment for a more extensive seedy-toe is to remove the outer crust of apparently healthy wall over the separation, clean up the area thoroughly, swab with strong tincture of iodine, and apply a Stockholm tar bandage which will need protection in some way. The bandage should be renewed from time to time. A more convenient way of protecting the exposed area is to cover it with a fluid rubber preparation or other special waterproof preparations which are available. The coronary band should receive attention to stimulate horn growth by rubbing with a stimulating liniment twice

189

a week or by application of a blister. Special shoeing is desirable to relieve pressure over the affected area.

SESAMOIDITIS

THE SESAMOID bones are two small, floating bones placed at the back of the fetlock joint in each limb. They are attached to the suspensory ligament and, with it, assist in keeping the lower end of the cannon bone in place on top of the sloping pastern bone, thus supporting the fetlock under stress.

Sesamoiditis is inflammation in the sesamoid region at the back of the fetlock joint, due to some injury either to the small bones, or to the ligaments and tendons associated therewith.

Cause

The condition may result from a blow, or from tearing of the attachments of the suspensory ligament to the sesamoid bones by strain or concussion, as may occur in jumping and, to a lesser degree, in flat racing.

Symptoms

Lameness and swelling at the back of the fetlock joint are the main symptoms. The swelling is hot and tender to the touch and the horse is inclined to walk on the toe. Diagnosis is not always easy and the condition is commonly mistaken for sprained fetlock or tendons.

Treatment

Sesamoiditis does not respond well to treatment, mainly because there is commonly tearing away of some of the fibres of the suspensory ligament from the sesamoid bones. The lameness may disappear with rest, only to return when the animal is worked. In the early stages, continuous cold water applications with a hose, or cold-water bandages, are helpful in relieving the pain and lameness. This may be followed by the application of an elastic adhesive bandage over a thick layer of cotton wool, the bandage extending from well below the fetlock joint to within a few inches of the knee or hock. Special shoes with high heels relieve pressure on the affected parts. When the acute stages have subsided, blistering or firing can be carried out and the horse given a long spell. Veterinary surgeons use corticosteroid therapy in the early stages of the disease.

SHOEING

THE SHOEING of horses which work on hard ground is a necessary evil. Many foot troubles will be avoided if the following rules are observed as nearly as possible when shoeing a horse:

190

1. Bring the wall of the foot down to what it would be if natural wear had occurred.
2. Fit the shoe to the outline of the foot, as rasping the outside of the wall makes it weak and brittle.
3. Never run the rasp over the outside of the wall, as it has a waterproof coat to keep in the necessary moisture and to keep out external moisture.
4. A sole cannot be too thick; it is there to protect the inner foot.
5. The bars should not be cut away; they are weight carriers, and the shoe should rest on them.
6. The frog should not be cut away; it is a cushion whose strength and function depend on it being level with the ground surface of the shoe.
7. The shoe should have a true and level bearing on the wall and bars.

An excellent little book, *Elements of Horseshoeing,* by J. A. Springhall, M.B.E., B.V.Sc., is available from University of Queensland Press, St. Lucia, Brisbane, Queensland.

SHOEING PRICKS

LAMENESS commonly occurs from a shoeing nail having been driven too close to or into the "quick" (*sensitive laminae*). An expert farrier knows at once when this has happened, but an amateur horse-shoer may continue to drive the nail right in.

Symptoms

If the nail has pricked the sensitive laminae, lameness follows soon after shoeing. If, as is often the case, the nail has been driven too close, so that it causes pressure on, but does not prick the sensitive laminae, lameness may not be shown for up to a week afterwards. The latter condition is known as "nail-binding" and results in a bulging of the horn on to the soft structures, causing a bruise and inflammation due to the pressure. The offending nail can usually be detected by pressure with pincers or by gently tapping with a light hammer over each nail. If this is unsuccessful, the hoof should be washed and brushed with soap and water and dried. Then the shoe should be carefully removed, drawing each nail separately and examining them for evidence of blood-stain or dampness, and observing whether there is any discharge from the nail hole. The nails may not be moist and there may be no discharge observed if the horse has only been shod two or three days, but from three to five days after shoeing some pus is usually seen, and this will be more copious if the horse has been shod for a longer period.

The pain caused by these wounds is great. The horse rests the foot on the toe, raises and lowers the leg or holds it from the ground, flexes the leg and knuckles at the fetlock. Swelling of the fetlock and back tendons is frequently seen, and the foot is found to be hot.

Treatment

If the nail prick is detected during shoeing, the offending nail should be withdrawn immediately, and the nail track treated with tincture of iodine or other suitable antiseptic. Another nail should not be driven in that place. If discovered later, the shoe should be removed in the manner described above, the offending nail detected, and the foot then soaked in a bucket of hot water to soften the horn and relieve pain. If the lameness is due to "nail-binding" and there is no evidence of infection, a few days of repeated soaking may overcome the condition. Paring down the sole in the vicinity of the nail hole can be carried out to relieve pressure. If, however, there is evidence of infection and pus formation, it will be necessary, after paring, to cut down over the nail hole, or at the site where pain is greatest on pressure, to permit of free discharge. The wound should be syringed with a weak antiseptic solution.

The foot can now, with advantage, be immersed in a bucket of warm water to which some antiseptic, or 2 tablespoons of salt, has been added. The surgical opening must be kept free until all discharge has ceased, and the area protected with a pad of cotton wool or tow, soaked in antiseptic, and held in place by an improvised boot. A good plan is to tack the shoe back lightly and to slip a piece of tin under the inner edges of the shoe to keep the pad in place. This also facilitates subsequent dressings. A warm kaolin poultice may also be applied in a similar manner. Any horse which has sustained a nail prick of the sensitive laminae should receive an injection of tetanus antitoxin. Neglected nail punctures, or those which have not been thoroughly treated, often lead to spread of infection within the foot and other complications. Veterinarians use antibiotics to control the infection.

SHOULDER LAMENESS

SHOULDER lameness is not as common a condition as is sometimes thought, and many suspected cases of lameness in the shoulder are found to be due to injuries lower down the limb, such as navicular disease, and foot injuries. Nevertheless, there are genuine shoulder lamenesses. Sprain of tendons, muscles and ligaments, and inflammation of the shoulder joint occur. Injury of the suprascapular nerve results in a bulging of the shoulder and may be the cause of muscular atrophy or wasting, commonly called "sweeny".

Causes

Amongst the causes of shoulder lameness are a fall, accompanied by violent concussion; a mis-step following a quick muscular effort; a jump with faulty landing; a slip on a wet, smooth road and collision with another horse or other object.

Symptoms

The diagnosis of shoulder lameness is sometimes difficult, and, although some of the symptoms of shoulder lameness are fairly definite, care is necessary not to confuse the suspected lameness in this region with trouble elsewhere in the limb. Lameness is more marked when the shoulder joint is involved than when the muscles alone are affected. Broadly, shoulder lameness is diagnosed by a restricted movement of the scapula (shoulder blade), marked lifting of the head as the limb is advanced, and a short step. The peculiar manner in which the leg is brought forward for another step in the act of walking or trotting is, in some instances, characteristic of injuries to the shoulder. The leg is brought forward with a bending round-swinging motion, and a shortening in the extension of the step. Lameness is often worse when travelling over soft ground, in contra-distinction to foot lameness, when it is lessened. The foot is carried close to the ground due to the shoulder being insufficiently raised and stumbling is frequent, especially on uneven ground. Lameness is often worse when the horse is trotted uphill. When backed, the horse will often drag the foot of the affected limb.

Atrophy or wasting of the muscles of the shoulder should not be diagnosed immediately as injury to the suprascapular nerve, because it may be due to inactivity of the animal and disuse of the shoulder muscles because of a painful condition elsewhere in the leg.

Treatment

Rest from work is the most important part of the treatment of shoulder lameness. Cold water applications from a hose, alternated with hot, wet blankets, are of value. Repeated massage over the affected area and the use of a mild liniment will be found beneficial. Obstinate cases may require blistering. When under veterinary care, diathermy is used to advantage. It is advisable to rest the horse in a loose box or shed with plenty of straw for a few days to a week and then turn it out in a paddock where it will obtain gentle exercise. If this is not possible, the horse should be given walking exercise on firm, even ground.

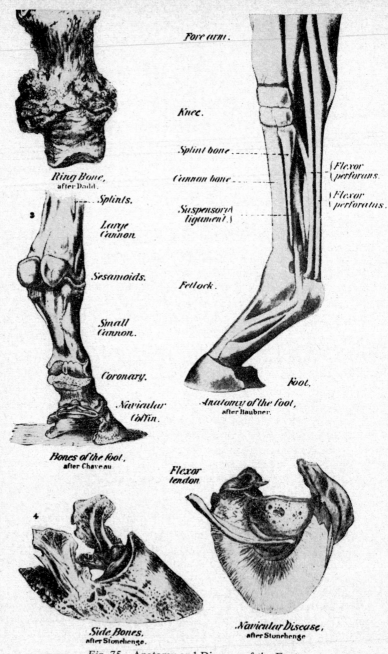

Fore arm.

Knee.

Splint bone

Cannon bone

{ Flexor
{ perforans.

{ Flexor
{ perforatus.

Suspensory
ligament.

Ring Bone,
after Dadd.

Splints.

Large
Cannon

Fetlock.

Sesamoids.

Small
Cannon.

Coronary.

Navicular
Coffin.

Bones of the foot,
after Chaveau

Anatomy of the foot,
after Haubner.

Foot.

Flexor
tendon

Side Bones,
after Stonehenge.

Navicular Disease,
after Stonehenge

Fig. 75   Anatomy and Diseases of the Foot.

(From Diseases of the Horse,
United States Department of Agriculture)

194

SIDEBONE

ATTACHED to the wings of the pedal bone (coffin bone) within the hoof, and extending above the hoof at the coronet, are the lateral cartilages. These cartilages, one on each side of each foot, are normally very resilient, forming a shock-absorbing apparatus within the hoof. The formation of bone within these cartilages produces sidebones. Hardening of the cartilages has the effect of cramping the structures of the internal part of the foot and may eventually lead to lameness, although this is not common. Sidebones are especially frequent in draught types of horses and are not so prone to occur in light horses. They occur chiefly in the front feet and are usually bilateral.

Cause

Although heredity plays a part in the development of sidebone, it is now considered that ossification of the lateral cartilages is a normal physiological process in the horse, especially in certain breeds. There are, however, a great many horses and ponies in which sidebone does not occur. Partial sidebone may occur in horses as they advance in age, and become complete in old age. Repeated concussion upon the pedal bone to which the cartilage is attached undoubtedly plays a part in the causation of sidebone, whilst contracted heels, ringbone, navicular disease, punctured wounds of the foot, quarter cracks, and even laminitis can be contributing causes.

Symptoms

In many instances, sidebones are of slow growth and, being usually unaccompanied by acute inflammation, they cause no lameness until, because of their size, they interfere with the action of the joint. In the earlier stages of the condition there may be slight inflammation, when heat can be detected over the seat of the affected cartilage, and there will be slight lameness, which later disappears. Since the deposit of bony matter often begins in that part of the cartilage where it is attached to the pedal bone, the diseased process may exist for some time before it can be felt or seen. Later on, however, the cartilage can be felt to have lost its elastic character, and by standing in front of the animal a prominence of the coronary region at the quarters can be seen.

Treatment

Should there be lameness in the early stages of the disease, this can be relieved by frequent soaking of the foot in cold water or by the use of cold water bandages. The treatment for later lameness, which may occur when the hoof is contracted, consists of lowering

o

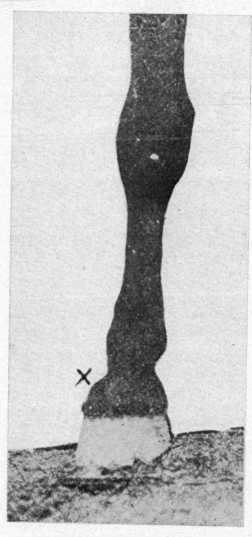

Fig. 76 Sidebone at X.

(*United States Department of Agriculture*)

196

the heels (to allow good frog pressure), thinning the horn of the hoof below the sidebone with a rasp and applying a blister to the coronary region on the affected side. This allows expansion of the hoof, with relief of pressure within the hoof. Special shoeing can be carried out to expand the hoof. A veterinary surgeon can do more by an operation. Many horses have sidebones without causing them any inconvenience, particularly if they work on soft ground.

SITFAST

A SITFAST is a form of dry gangrene, resulting from pressure on a circumscribed area of the skin, with firm adherence of the dead tissue to the living tissue below. The horny slough may involve the superficial part of the skin only, or the whole thickness of the skin, and even some of the structures beneath. Sitfasts occur as a result of pressure by badly fitting harness or by irritating masses of dirt, sweat and hairs under the harness. They are most common under the saddle.

Treatment consists of cutting out the dead irritating slough with a sharp knife, following which the area is treated as an open wound with antiseptics and antibiotic dressings. If the fascia or bone has become necrotic, the dead portion must be removed. The surgical treatment should be performed by a veterinarian. The horse must be spelled until the wound has healed or the saddle and harness adjusted so that no pressure comes on the affected parts.

For further information, see *Saddle Galls*.

SKIN DISEASES

See *Eczema, Lice, Mange, Nettlerash, Photosensitization, Queensland Itch, Ringworm*

SLEEPY FOAL DISEASE (Shigellosis)

THIS IS an acute, highly-fatal, septicaemic disease of new-born foals, caused by an organism now known as *Actinobacillus equuli*, but formerly as *Shigella equirulis*. This organism is common in the intestinal tract and tissues of normal mares, in which it does not cause disease.

Because foals may be observed sick at birth, or within a few hours and up to three days of birth, it would appear that infection of the foal occurs in the uterus of the mare, but could occur through the navel after birth. The disease is responsible for the deaths of many young foals in most countries, including Australia. The symptoms are

197

sleepiness, lethargy, prostration, high fever, diarrhoea, rapid respiration, and the foal ceasing to suck its mother.

Many foals die within twelve to twenty-four hours. Those that survive the acute stage of the disease develop inflammation of the joints and abscesses of the muscles, and are lame. The latter animals usually die within a week, when post-mortem examination shows abscesses in the kidneys and elsewhere.

Owing to the rapid onset of the symptoms and the development of septicaemia, treatment is difficult and calls for the early administration of specific antibiotics and supportive treatment by a veterinarian.

The disease might be prevented by the prophylactic administration of various antibiotics at birth, by dusting the navel cord with sulphanilamide powder, or applying a suitable weak antiseptic solution, and by general hygienic precautions at foaling time.

SORE BACKS

See *Saddle Galls*

SORE SHINS (Periostitis, Ostitis)

"SORE SHINS" is the term given to acute inflammation of the front of the large cannon bone of the foreleg. The same condition is sometimes seen on the front of the cannon bone of the hind leg. The trouble occurs more commonly in young horses when first put to work, especially in race-horses during the early weeks of training.

Because of the close connection between the *periosteum* (covering membrane of the bone) and the bone itself, it is very difficult to determine whether an *ostitis* (inflammation of the bone) is also present. This has a bearing on the result of any treatment carried out.

Causes

In young horses, concussion appears to be the most important causative factor, because the symptoms are observed after exercise. In older horses, external violence is mainly responsible for the condition, although it may be due to inflammation of a ligament or tendon spreading to the *periosteum* of the cannon bone. Severe forms of the condition may be associated with bacterial activity.

Symptoms

In young animals, there is a hot, painful swelling in the front of one or both large cannon bones of the fore legs, and, much less frequently, of those of the hind legs. Lameness is present and the horse walks with a short stride. The swelling subsequently thickens,

198

when the heat and pain are less. In older horses the area is very tender to the touch, but the heat and swelling seen in young animals is usually not present.

Treatment

Rest is essential until all soreness and inflammation have disappeared. The acute inflammation may be relieved by cold packs or by hosing the affected legs. Subsequently, hot fomentations should be given and an astringent liniment applied. *Antiphlogistine*, a proprietary preparation, will be found useful, lightly bandaged over the affected areas. Still later, iodine ointment can be used. In those cases where the swelling persists and exostosis (bony growths) appear, blistering might be carried out to advantage.

SPAVIN

SPAVIN means a disease of the hock of a horse, of which there are two common types,

1. Bone spavin, and
2. Bog spavin.

BONE SPAVIN

This occurs in two forms, true or "jack" spavin, and occult or hidden spavin. True bone spavin might be described simply as a chronic arthritis, which results in the union of the small bones at the inner and lower part of the hock, so that they become a solid mass. The enlargement caused by the exostosis (abnormal outgrowth of bone) is usually greatest on the inner side of the joint. It may be most easily observed by comparing the hocks one with another, standing outside each foreleg in turn to look at the inner sides of the hocks; or it may be felt by the hand.

Occult spavin is an arthritis of the articular surfaces (joints) of the hock bones, or between the hock bones and the cannon bone, but there are no visible bony outgrowths as seen in true bone spavin. It can only be diagnosed from evidence of pain in the hock joint and limitation of hock flexion in the affected leg.

Causes

There are a number of suggested causes of bone spavin, including faulty hock conformation; hereditary predisposition; injury or overexertion as in jumping, more particularly in young horses when not trained or when out of condition; excessive concussion, as occurs in horses trotted on hard roads; and mineral deficiency.

Bone spavin affects all classes and ages of horses from two-year-olds onwards. It would appear that concussion is generally one of the main causes of spavin.

Symptoms

In true bone spavin, the higher and more forward the bony outgrowths occur on the hock the greater is the possibility of severe lameness, because in such cases there is more likely to be interference with the action of the joint than if the outgrowths were at the side. Bone spavin usually develops gradually and lameness may be noticed before there is any bony enlargement. In early cases of both types the lameness is noticed first thing in the morning, disappears after the horse has "warmed-up", only to return again after rest. This characteristic becomes less marked as the disease advances and

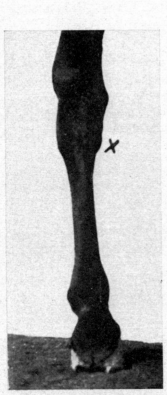
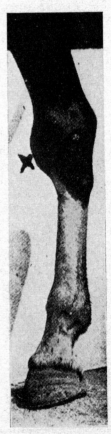

Fig. 77 Bone Spavin at X.
(*United States Department of Agriculture*)

Fig. 78 Bog Spavin at X.
(*United States Department of Agriculture*)

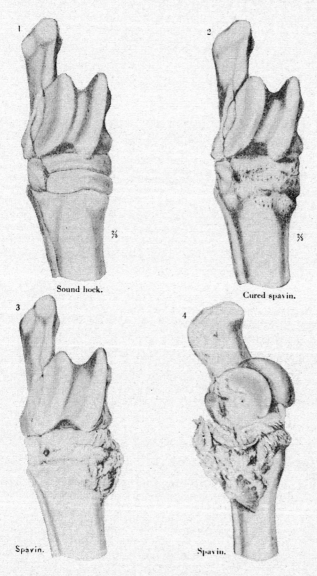

1 Sound hock.

2 Cured spavin.

3 Spavin.

4 Spavin.

Fig. 79 Bone Spavin.

(From Diseases of the Horse,
United States Department of Agriculture)

201

lameness becomes more constant. As the disease progresses the horse tends to drag the toe, consequently the toe of the shoe or hoof shows signs of wear. When standing, the horse is inclined to rest the toe on the ground with the heel slightly raised.

A well-recognized test for bone spavin, although not infallible, is to lift the affected leg from the ground, holding the foot high so that the cannon bone is against the gaskin for one to two minutes, and then have the horse trotted as soon as the leg is released. The lameness will then be greatly intensified and so assist in diagnosis. A comparison should be made with the other hock.

Treatment

A long rest of about six months is most important in the treatment of bone spavin. In the early stages, cold water applications by continued hosing may assist in arresting the progress of the inflammation. In the case of valuable horses, where expense has not to be considered, a prolonged course of diathermy may bring about good results. Maintaining the balance of the foot by cutting down the toe, leaving as much heel as possible, and perhaps putting heel calkins on the shoe, are also recommended. Fusion of some of the bones of the hock usually takes place, and once the bones have grown firmly together, lameness disappears and the horse may not be seriously incapacitated in its work. Thus, if the progress of the disease cannot be arrested early, and this is commonly the case, serviceability rather than soundness is the aim of treatment.

Point firing over a bone spavin followed by blistering has, in the past, been commonly used to hasten ankylosis of the bones of the hock, with the idea of prolonging the usefulness of the horse. It is not now so commonly carried out. It should be remembered that the arthritic condition is progressive and will continue even after ankylosis has occurred.

BOG SPAVIN

This is a distension of the synovial bursa ("oil-bag") of the hock at the inner and upper part of the joint and is similar to a windgall. The condition is seen more commonly in horses that have straight or upright hocks. It also occurs in young horses which are overworked.

Causes

Although bog spavin is often regarded as indicating inherited weakness of the hock joint, the condition is frequently seen in aged stallions and breeding mares with well-shaped joints, when it is due to strain of the hocks. In young horses, it may be due to the greater elasticity of the joint structures and result from slipping backwards

202

with the hind legs. Actually bog spavin is a chronic synovitis of the joint, brought about by wear, hard work, or accident.

Symptoms

The condition appears as a soft, fluctuating swelling about one-third the way down on the front and towards the inside of the hock. It is usually not hot to the touch and does not cause lameness. In other cases the swelling is at first hard, painful to the touch and accompanied by lameness, but this is not common. In the main, bog spavin does not cause lameness unless the condition is complicated by inflammation and bone involvement, and therefore rarely interferes with the usefulness of the horse. It does, of course, constitute an unsightly blemish.

Treatment

Although bog spavin is usually not a serious condition and sometimes disappears without any form of treatment, it should not be regarded lightly. Rest is an essential part of treatment. If there is no heat in the swelling and there is no lameness, it is unwise to attempt to reduce the size of the swelling, the best treatment being to turn the horse out into a well-grassed paddock. When the part is hot, indicating inflammation, and there is lameness, hot fomentations are indicated. When the inflammation has subsided, a pressure bandage with cotton wool, if correctly adjusted, often has a good effect. A cooling astringent lotion should be used with the bandage. Compression is sometimes achieved by means of an elastic bandage. Repeated application of tincture of iodine, once or twice daily, has been found useful in reducing an early case of bog spavin, but is of little value for one of long standing. In those cases which do not respond to rest and these simple treatments, the excess fluid in the joint capsule can be aspirated and a corticosteroid injected by a veterinarian. Diathermy treatment can also be given.

The condition has a tendency to recur.

SPEEDY-CUT

SPEEDY-CUT is the name given to an injury on the inner surface of the lower part of the knee, caused by the horse striking it with the inner portion of the shoe of the opposite foot, at fast pace.

Horses with faulty leg or foot conformation, or those which are very tired, especially if forced over rough ground, are most likely to sustain the injury. There may or may not be an actual cut in the skin, but in any case the bruise which results can be serious and the pain caused may bring the horse down. The leg swells and is very painful. When the blow is often repeated, as is common, a permanent enlargement remains.

Treatment and Prevention

Hot fomentations, followed by the application of a cold water bandage, are recommended for a fresh speedy-cut. If the skin is cut, it should be treated as an open wound with mild antiseptics (see *Wound Treatment*).

To prevent speedy-cutting, shoe the opposite foot as close as possible at the inside toe and quarter, rasping off some of the wall if necessary, and rounding off the lower edge of the web of the shoe. Special speedy-cutting boots, or a pad of felt or rubber on the inner side of the shoe of the striking foot may be required.

When buying a riding horse, it is important to look and feel for old scars or enlargements from previous injuries.

A horse which continually "speedy-cuts" is dangerous to the rider.

SPLINTS

A SPLINT is a bony outgrowth between the cannon bone and one or both of the small "splint bones". These are found on each side of the rear surface of the cannon bones of the fore and hind legs, and extend from the knee or hock to about the lower third of the main bone. The bony outgrowth results from inflammation of the fibrous membrane covering the bone, or of the ligamentous attachment between the cannon and the splint bone.

Young horses are most prone to splints, which occur more commonly on the forelegs and usually on the inside of the leg. Occasionally they appear on the outside of the leg. At times splints are found on the outside and inside of the hind legs.

During evolutionary processes, the horse developed from a five-toed animal into one which moved on a greatly modified and developed structure corresponding to the original middle claw. Instead of walking with the claw flat on the ground, it eventually walked on the point, and this became enclosed in a hoof. In the process, most of the other bones disappeared.

In the animal we know, the knee corresponds to the wrist, and the hock to the heel of the human, and the main bones below that have developed only from the central one of the original five.

Just below the knee and the hock, on each side of the cannon bones, a remnant remains of the two adjoining bones. These are known as the splint bones. They form part of the joint with the knee or hock,

204

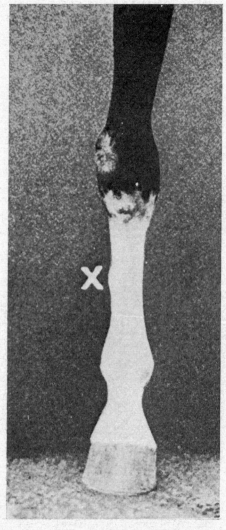

Fig. 80   Splint at X.
(United States Department of Agriculture)

but gradually diminish in size until they disappear about two-thirds of the way down the cannon bone.

In the young horse, the shafts of the splint bones are attached to the cannon bone by a ligament, which is gradually replaced by bone as the horse ages.

Strain on the joining ligament in young horses is the most common cause of trouble, but if this period is passed safely, the development of splints is not as likely.

Causes

In the majority of cases, the bony deposit known as a "splint" appears at the junction of the splint bone and the cannon bone—usually in young horses, before bony union has taken place between these bones. Sprain of the ligamentous attachment between the cannon bone and the splint bone, or injury to the membranous covering of the bone, is likely to give rise to an exostosis of bony material—a splint. Sometimes the exostosis is confined to the cannon bone, when it is usually due to a blow.

Fast movement on hard ground causes repeated concussion effects through the column of bones between the knee and the fetlock, and is a common cause of splints. The condition occurs quite commonly during the training of young horses or when they are first put to heavy work. Jumping is also a cause of splints, not so much because of striking the leg against a rail or fence, but from the concussion of landing on the other side of the hurdle. Horses with poor conformation, and bad action, are likely to strike themselves, producing mechanical damage leading to splints. The hind legs are much less exposed to the effects of concussion than the forelegs. Splints on the hind legs, when they do occur, seldom cause much trouble.

Deficiency or imbalance of dietary minerals may cause young horses to be more susceptible to stresses leading to splint formation.

Symptoms

Lameness may occur before any swelling appears on the bone. Careful examination should be made along the inside and the outside of the cannon bone for evidence of tenderness under pressure with the fingers. To examine a limb for splints, the knee or hock should be flexed with the cannon bone parallel to the ground and, with the thumb on one side and the fingers on the other side, pressed evenly from the knee downwards along the junction of the large and small bones. When splints are forming, a slight swelling may be felt. The inflamed part will be hot, and the animal will show pain by snatching the leg away when the part is pressed. A hind leg may be similarly examined.

Horses with splints may walk normally, but be lame at the trot. Lameness increases with exercise. The bony enlargements, which appear some time after lameness is shown, may develop to the size of a pea or a walnut and are sometimes of a longish and irregular form. The lameness occasioned by a recently-formed splint is in no way proportional to the size of the bony outgrowth. Small splints often cause severe lameness, while large ones sometimes occasion little or no inconvenience. There are a number of reasons for this, associated with the extent of the inflammatory processes, but the seriousness of splints depends mainly on their location. A splint which does not interfere with a joint, tendon, ligament or nerve, causes lameness only during the period of formation. When splints are near the knee or hock joints, or touching the back tendons, they are very troublesome.

Treatment

In foals and yearlings, splints often disappear spontaneously, and treatment of these young animals should not be hurried. The mineral intake of the young horses should be checked and deficiencies or imbalance corrected. Rest is an essential part of treatment for splints and the lameness resulting therefrom, but a little regular walking exercise is desirable. This is best obtained if the animal can be turned out into a well-grassed paddock where it will obtain sufficient exercise while grazing. Reduction of recent splints can be assisted by massage twice a day and the application of a pressure bandage. When massaging the splint, a little olive oil should be used to prevent soreness of the skin. To apply a pressure bandage, use a light cotton wool pad or a piece of sole leather or thick rubber enclosed in cotton wool and bind this firmly over the splint. If reduction of the splint has not occurred and lameness still persists, after a month or six weeks of this treatment, the application of a mild counter-irritant may produce a good effect. A useful preparation is biniodide of mercury, 1 in 16, applied over the splint and gently rubbed in for five minutes once weekly for several weeks. The horse should be spelled during the treatment and the return to work should be made very gradually. If the counter-irritant treatment proves to be ineffective, point firing and blistering by a veterinarian will be necessary.

Prominent splints on the inside of the leg, which may be repeatedly knocked by the opposite leg, can be removed by operation.

If a horse is under six years of age, splints should be looked upon as likely to cause trouble, a fact which should be considered when buying a horse. If the horse is over six years old, splints can be discounted unless lameness is present. Even if a large bony outgrowth occurs on the cannon bone and the horse is sound, it is preferable to put up with the blemish rather than to attempt some drastic home method of removing it, which may perhaps leave a worse blemish. Many horses are permanently injured or badly blemished by ill-advised attempts on the part of owners to reduce splints. Particularly does this apply to the use of strong acids.

Finally, skilful shoeing is important to prevent striking and to effect a proper distribution of weight, thus preventing splints caused by mechanical injury.

SPRAIN OF TENDONS

See *Tendons—Sprained*

SPRUNG HOCK

THIS NAME, not now commonly used, refers to a severe sprain of the ligaments of the inner and back part of the hock, accompanied by other complications.

It occurs as the result of over-exertion of the joint as may occur when jumping, or from slipping on a wet surface. The ligaments may in this way be severely stretched and injured. The surface of the bones, where the ligaments are inserted, may become inflamed and a synovitis of the hock joint may also occur.

Symptoms

The symptoms vary according to the severity of the sprain of the ligaments and the possible involvement of tendons and bones. There is usually a good deal of swelling all round the hock, pronounced lameness, and the hock is carried stiffly, little or no weight being placed on the limb. At rest, the weight is placed on the toe of the foot. Pain is shown when the joint is manipulated.

Treatment

The treatment of acute cases comprises rest and the application of hot and cold water, gentle massage, stimulating liniments, and bandages. With such local treatment, and adequate rest, most cases recover. Should the condition become chronic, blistering, firing or other forms of treatment by a veterinarian will be necessary.

STAGGERS

SYMPTOMS of staggers, incoordination of movement and convulsions have many causes, including brain diseases and congestion due to an increased flow of blood to the brain.

When horses were commonly used for draught purposes, a condition known in stable language as "megrims" not uncommonly occurred, usually while the horse was in work and especially in hot weather. The symptoms shown were shivering, shaking of the head, staggers and the horse falling to the ground unconscious, but from which it rapidly recovered. Although the exact cause of this condition is still not understood, it was well recognized that horses working in an ordinary collar were most prone to attacks of megrims, which suggested that pressure of the collar gave rise to congestion of the brain. Although this may have been secondary to some other condition, it was observed that when such horses were worked with a breast strap, the trouble did not occur. A tightly-adjusted throat strap has also been held responsible for the condition. Occasionally a chronic form of this condition occurred, suggesting a symptomatic epilepsy. Local treatment for megrims consisted of douching the head with cold water and protecting the animal from the sun.

A disease known as *ataxia* in horses, which appears to be similar to a condition known in England as "grass staggers" and "grass sickness", has been recorded in the coastal districts of New South Wales and also in Queensland. Affected animals are dull and sleepy, show incoordination of gait and other symptoms. It has been postulated that the disease may be due to a virus, but some years ago a bowel toxin was isolated, suggesting that the disease may be enterotoxaemia.

Still another condition, referred to as equine sensory ataxia ("wobbles"), has been the subject of much research in the United States of America. The disease has occurred in New South Wales, where it has also been investigated. In this disease there is also incoordination of gait, associated with degeneration of the spinal cord. The underlying cause has not yet been definitely established.

STIFLE LAMENESS

See *Displacement of the Patella*

STOMACH—RUPTURE OF

RUPTURE of the stomach is not a common condition in the horse. Nevertheless, it has occurred either from over-distension, when horses have been fed large quantities of bulky food, or have had unrestricted access to grain. It may also occur as a sequel to flatulent colic when there is great distension with gas, and has been known to occur following violent exertion such as jumping, or following a sudden fall when the stomach is distended with food or gas. Diseases of the

209

mucous membranes of the stomach, calculi ("stones") and tumours may also be responsible.

Symptoms

The general symptoms of distension of the stomach are colicky pains, which are not of much diagnostic value. Rapid and difficult breathing, sweating, trembling and staggering are common symptoms, and the horse may sit up like a dog for considerable periods and attempt to vomit. Actually some vomiting may occur, although this is difficult for the horse. The strong contractions of the abdominal muscles subject the stomach to severe pressure, which contributes to stomach rupture.

When the rupture has occurred, the attempts at vomiting cease and the horse is temporarily relieved. Cold patchy sweating and trembling continue, and there is severe congestion of the visible mucous membranes. The temperature, which is at first raised, becomes subnormal. A slimy food-stained liquid may come through the nostrils and mouth. Death follows in a few hours but may be delayed longer.

Treatment

There is, of course, no treatment for rupture of the stomach.

STONES IN THE KIDNEYS, URETERS AND BLADDER

See *Urinary Calculi*

STRANGLES

STRANGLES, referred to in the United States of America as "distemper", is an acute contagious disease of equines, namely the horse, ass and mule. It is characterized by fever, a catarrhal inflammation of the nasal cavities and throat, and the development of abscesses in the lymph glands, especially between the branches of the lower jaw. Young horses are most commonly affected, but horses of any age can contract the disease, especially those which have not previously had it. One attack usually confers immunity for life, but sometimes the immunity breaks down and the animal can suffer a second attack. Naturally, an epidemic of strangles is more likely to occur when a number of horses are kept together, such as on stud horse farms and riding schools. The disease caused much trouble in mounted units of the armed forces in both World Wars, but, although it can still be troublesome, it is now of minor importance in most countries.

Cause

An organism known as *Streptococcus equi* is considered to be the main cause of strangles and, although it may be associated with other organisms, *S. equi* is always present in the nasal discharges and pus during the course of the disease. Exposure to cold, over-work, poor feeding and other factors which lower the animal's resistance are predisposing causes of the disease.

Horses most commonly become infected from the nasal or pus discharges from infected horses which contaminate the feed and watering troughs and pasture. Infection can also occur by inhalation of droplets coughed or breathed out by infected animals. The portal of entry of the germs is through the mucous membranes of the nose and pharynx. Recently recovered animals can spread infection for at least four weeks after an attack.

The organism is fairly resistant to environmental influences. Stables which have housed diseased animals and in which discharges will have been coughed on to the floor, walls and into the manger are sources of infection. Likewise, harness, nosebags, grooming utensils and the clothes of attendants can spread the infection.

The period of incubation—the time from exposure to infection until the development of symptoms of the disease—is four to eight days.

Symptoms

The main symptoms shown in typical or uncomplicated cases of strangles are fever with temperature of 103 to 105° F., nasal catarrh, and swelling of the submaxillary lymph glands between the branches of the lower jaw, the pharyngeal (throat) lymph glands and sometimes the parotid lymph glands below the ear. There is often a varying degree of pharyngitis and laryngitis.

Attention is first drawn to the presence of the disease by a nasal discharge, difficulty in swallowing due to sore throat, cough, loss of appetite and general depression. The nasal discharge is at first watery but subsequently becomes thickened and pus-like. Within a few days, evidence of the germs having become arrested in the lymphatic glands about the head is shown by swelling of certain of these glands. Pus accumulates within the swollen glands which become hot and painful. In the course of another few days to a week, a soft fluctuating point is noticed at the peak of the swelling, and rupture of the abscess at this point commonly occurs. This is usually followed by a fall in temperature to normal, general improvement in the animal and, provided there are no complications, recovery in two to four weeks.

Atypical forms of strangles occur as a result of metastasis—a

211

P

spread from the original site of the disease—and abscess formation in other organs including the lungs, liver, spleen, kidneys, brain, and the mesenteric lymph glands in the peritoneal attachment of the intestines. When these occur, the symptoms vary a great deal, depending on the location of the abscesses. For example, an abscess in the lung is likely to result in acute pneumonia. When the mesenteric lymph glands are involved, there are symptoms of colic or general abdominal pain, constipation, loss of appetite and fluctuating temperature. Such animals fall away in condition and death may occur from peritonitis due to rupture of an internal abscess some weeks or months later.

Another atypical form of strangles, seen by me in army horses, shows typical strangles symptoms—nasal discharge, cough, fever and acute depression, without abscess formation.

Diseases likely to supervene on an attack of strangles are roaring and whistling, broken-wind and purpura haemorrhagica.

Treatment

Since strangles is a highly contagious disease, affected animals should be immediately isolated, and care taken that the disease is not spread to other horses by feeding utensils or the hands and clothing of the attendants. Complete rest and good nursing are important in treatment of an affected animal. No attempt should be made to drench the horse, since, owing to the difficulty of swallowing, there is a risk that some of the drench may pass to the lungs and cause a fatal pneumonia.

Provided the weather is not too cold, a horse not accustomed to being stabled is best left in the open in a small convenient paddock and kept warm by rugging. Feed should be given from a box on the ground, because the nasal discharges come away more freely when the horse has its nose well down while feeding. Clean drinking water should be provided and repeatedly changed before it becomes fouled with nasal discharges. Sponging of the nose and eyes will frequently prevent "scalding" of the skin and is part of the general care of the patient. Steaming of the horse's head three or four times a day, by holding the head over a bucket of hot water to which a little Friar's balsam has been added, will be found beneficial. Do not attempt to steam a horse's head in a bag.

Antibiotic and sulphonamide drugs are now used as standard treatment by veterinarians for strangles. The prompt and repeated use of these drugs will often prevent abscess formation and avoid the necessity for blistering and opening of superficial abscesses about the head. Where professional assistance is not available and suitable antibiotic treatment is not given, it is advisable to foment swollen lymphatic glands with hot water or to rub in a stimulating liniment, but preferably to rub in a mild blistering ointment, obtainable from any chemist, to hasten "ripening" of the abscess. Before applying the blister, place a ring of petroleum jelly or something similar right around the swollen gland. This will prevent the blister from "running" and scalding the skin in other places. When the abscess points, it should be lanced, as it is desirable to release the pus as soon as possible. The best way for a non-professional person to do this is to pass the blade of a sharp pocket knife, which has previously been sterilized, through a cork, having the blade projecting about half to three-quarters of an inch. The blade is plunged into the soft part of the abscess up to the cork, and a downward stroke made. A fairly large opening is necessary, not less than an inch long, both to permit of adequate drainage of the abscess and to prevent the edges of the wound healing before the abscess has completely discharged. The abscess cavity should be well syringed out daily with some weak antiseptic solution, such as *Cetavlon* or *Dettol* and water, or a tea-spoonful of salt in a pint of boiled water. This also helps to prevent the wound healing before all pus has been discharged.

Every endeavour should be made to get the horse to eat. If the animal can swallow easily, chopped green feed should be fed if natural grazing is not available. Steamed hay, crushed oats and sliced carrots are tempting feeds. Where swallowing is difficult, sloppy foods are more easily and safely taken, such as thin oatmeal or linseed gruels and an occasional bran mash.

A working horse should be given a month's spell after an attack of strangles.

Prevention

Horses can be vaccinated for the prevention of strangles. Whilst not always conferring an absolute immunity, this reduces the severity of the disease should it occur.

STRINGHALT

STRINGHALT is an obscure condition in the horse in which there is an involuntary movement of one or both hind legs. The foot is suddenly and spasmodically lifted from the ground much higher than it is normally carried, with excessive flexion of the leg, sometimes up to the belly. Cases of the condition occurring in the foreleg have been recorded, but are extremely rare. The disease does not seem to be influenced by the horse's age, young and old horses of any breed being affected, but the condition does seem to become worse with age.

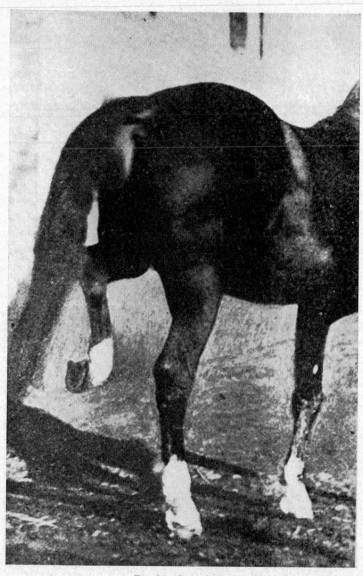

Fig. 81   Stringhalt.
(*United States Department of Agriculture*)

Cause

There has been much theorizing as to the cause of true stringhalt, but the actual cause is very much in doubt. It has been suggested that the seat of the trouble is in the spinal cord, or that it may be due to degeneration of the sciatic or peroneal nerves.

Symptoms

The first manifestations of the condition are sometimes very slight. It may be noticeable when the horse is backed out of a stable when cold, or on turning the animal round to one side and then to the other. Again, it may be apparent only at the trot, or at a walk, and at other times only when the animal is turned around.

The usefulness of the horse may not be greatly diminished when mildly affected with stringhalt, but, as the peculiar action interferes with movement, the condition must be classified as an unsoundness. The constant concussion resulting from the horse striking the ground violently with the foot may lead to other complications.

Treatment

Certain operations, including peroneal tenotomy, are performed by veterinarians to render the horse more serviceable, otherwise no treatment is of much avail.

AUSTRALIAN STRINGHALT

What is known as Australian stringhalt occurs quite frequently in some areas of Australia under certain seasonal conditions—usually in midsummer. It has been seen in the central western district of New South Wales and has been recorded elsewhere in Australia and in New Zealand.

The symptoms are similar to true stringhalt, the flexing of the hind legs being even greater than in the latter condition. Quite a number of horses in a locality may be affected. Fortunately, most of these cases are of a temporary nature and after a few weeks or months the animals recover. On the other hand, in certain recorded outbreaks quite a large proportion of the horses have remained permanently incapacitated.

Various plants have been suspected as being responsible for the condition, but nothing definite has been proved by feeding trials carried out at the laboratory or in the field. It has been shown, however, that if a horse affected with Australian stringhalt is moved to another district, recovery usually occurs.

SUMMER SORES—CUTANEOUS HABRONEMIASIS

See *Parasites—Stomach Worms*

SUNSTROKE

See *Heat Stroke*

SUPERPURGATION

SUPERPURGATION is excessive purgation or diarrhoea that is at times induced by the action of some purgative medicine. It may be accompanied by inflammation of the bowels, when it is serious.

Cause

Although, in rare instances, superpurgation follows a correct dose of purgative medicine, it is most likely to result under the following circumstances: too large a dose of purgative medicine; the administration of purgative medicines to a horse suffering from respiratory or other debilitating diseases; riding or driving a horse when purging; allowing the animal to drink large quantities of cold water while the purgative medicine is working; exposure to cold wet conditions during purging.

A condition of superpurgation can also occur in animals poisoned by irritant chemicals and some plants, and also in severe cases of enteric infections.

Symptoms

Diarrhoea persisting for a longer period than it should after a dose of purgative medicine. Additional symptoms include dejection, loss of appetite, colicky pains, coldness of the extremities, accelerated breathing, weakness and marked thirst.

Treatment

Because superpurgation may terminate fatally following inflammation of the bowels, professional assistance should be obtained. It is a common practice after a horse has purged from twelve to twenty-four hours after medicine, to feed dry oats and hay. 1 oz. of chlorodyne in a quart of rice or starch water may be given to advantage and can be repeated after two hours if necessary. The horse should be kept warm by rugging, and allowed a limited amount of water to drink, preferably luke-warm water in small quantities. Oatmeal or wheat flour gruel are useful drinks. Brandy and port wine in doses of 2 to 4 oz. may be given several times a day.

Laminitis ("founder") is a not infrequent sequel to superpurgation and can be guarded against by removing the shoes and standing the horse in water or on wet sawdust or straw.

SUPPRESSION OF URINE

SUPPRESSION of urine in horses takes place when, for some reason or other, the urine is not secreted by the kidneys. It may arise from a heart condition affecting the general circulation of the blood, or from functional derangement of the kidneys. It is not the same as retention of urine in the bladder.

The horse makes frequent attempts to urinate and only succeeds in passing very small quantities of urine. The bladder, which can be palpated by the hand and arm in the rectum, will be found to be empty.

Prompt attention by a veterinarian is essential, as the real cause of the trouble must first be ascertained before any attempt is made at treatment. For example, if the trouble arises from the effects of inflammation of the kidneys, the use of diuretic drugs would be harmful.

RETENTION OF URINE

This is mentioned here so that it may be contrasted with suppression of urine.

In retention, the urine is secreted normally by the kidneys and passes along the ureters (tubes from the kidneys) to the bladder, but is not ejected.

There are many causes of retention of urine, such as spasm of the neck of the bladder, which could be caused by the application of a cantharadies blister to a large surface of the body; paralysis of the muscles of the bladder; enlargement of the glands near the neck of the bladder; or the presence of calculi ("stones") in the bladder or in the urethral passage. When a horse has been working hard over a long period and has not been given the opportunity to urinate, spasm of the neck of the bladder sometimes occurs and the horse is unable to urinate fully although he is anxious to do so.

The distended condition of the bladder can be felt by rectal examination.

Enemas of warm water, followed by gentle pressure on the bladder by the hand in the rectum, will frequently cause the horse to urinate. If this treatment is not successful, the urine must be removed by a catheter.

Other conditions, such as calculi, require special treatment.

See also *Kidneys—Inflammation of*, *Colic* and *Calculi*

TEETH—IRREGULARITIES OF MOLARS

MOLAR teeth are required both to cut and to grind the feed. The bearing surfaces of the upper and lower teeth are worn by the movements of the jaws so that they meet with a surface which slopes downwards and outwards. This results in the formation of a sharp edge along the outer border of the upper teeth and the inner border of the lower teeth. These edges are kept sharp by the grinding of the teeth and such sharpness must not be regarded as abnormal. Sometimes, however, due to malformation of the jaws, softness of the teeth or the direction of the teeth, there may be abnormal wear and sharp projections occur which can abrade or cut the tongue and cheeks. The bottom last molars sometimes grow up behind the top ones and penetrate the jaw. Injuries to other molar teeth may cause them to have broken sharp edges. Evidence of such irregularities of the molar teeth is usually shown by the horse "quidding" its feed, or slobbering while feeding. Sometimes there may be evidence of pain during mastication, the head being held to one side while chewing. A horse being ridden may pull to one side and toss the head if there are sharp projections or edges on the front premolars, as these may abrade the cheeks or tongue from the action of the bit.

Irregularities of the molar teeth can be discovered by backing the horse into a corner, grasping the tongue with the left hand and using the tip of the tongue as a gag against the upper jaw. The back

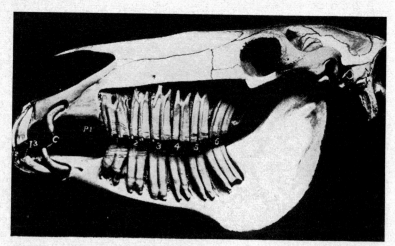

Fig. 82　Skull of Horse, five years old, Sculptured to Show Embedded Parts
of Teeth.

(*From Sisson-Grossman: Anatomy of the Domestic Animals, 4th edition.
Philadelphia, W. B. Saunders Co., 1953*)

teeth may now be looked at or felt with safety. A mouth-gag, of course, facilitates an examination of the mouth.

Molar teeth may be rasped if they have unduly sharp edges or projections, or minor irregularities on the table surfaces which are incompatible with the opposing teeth. It is preferable to have a veterinary surgeon do this, to ensure that it is carried out correctly. General irregularity of the molars in old age is not as common as is generally supposed, and, in the past, there has been much unnecessary filing of teeth.

Misplaced or malformed teeth should be extracted by a veterinarian.

See also *Dentition* and *Ageing*

TEMPERATURE, PULSE AND RESPIRATION

TEMPERATURE

The normal temperature of the horse averages 100° F., varying from 99·5 to 100·5° F. (37·5 to 38° C.). The temperature is taken in the rectum with an ordinary human clinical thermometer, preferably one with a stub end, and it should be held in the rectum for at least double the time indicated on its register (one to two minutes). The thermometer should be shaken down below the normal temperature, then wetted or oiled to make its passage easy, and passed through the anus into the rectum and held there. It is important that the bulb of the thermometer be kept in contact with the rectal lining. If the horse is restless, an assistant should hold up a front foot.

The normal temperature of the horse varies somewhat under different conditions. It is higher in foals and yearlings, which may register up to 102° F., and is higher after severe exercise or in very hot weather. Generally, it is not greatly affected by average climatic variations.

A rise of temperature to 102·5° F. indicates a mild fever; if it reaches 104° F., the fever is moderate; 106° F. is a high fever, and above this it is regarded as very high.

Before putting the thermometer away, wash it in water or cold antiseptic solution and shake the mercury down.

PULSE

The pulse rate of the healthy adult horse varies from 30 to 40 per minute, but is much higher in young animals, being up to 70 per minute in foals. The pulse may be counted and its character may be determined at any point where a large artery is close to the skin and passes over a hard surface such as a bone, cartilage or tendon. A convenient place is at the angle of the jaw where an artery crosses the bone. Its throb can be felt just before it turns around the lower border of the jawbone. The pulse may also be taken inside the fore-arm at the level of the elbow joint, where an artery crosses immediately over the bone.

The first and second fingers should be pressed lightly on the skin over the artery.

The animal should be at perfect rest when the pulse is taken, as exercise and excitement quicken it. Experience is necessary to obtain important information from the pulse rate. It is faster in fevers and slower and weaker in non-febrile debilitating diseases. The pulse rate and its character (whether it is stronger or weaker than it should be) is important in the diagnosis of disease, especially when considered together with other diagnostic aids, such as temperature and respiration.

RESPIRATION

The normal respiration of a six-year-old, healthy horse, observed by viewing the flank movements, is 8 to 12 inspirations per minute. It is usual to count the inspirations for half a minute and then to double the result. The respiration rate is greater in young horses and may be up to 14 or 15 inspirations per minute.

The type of respiration is very important in the diagnosis of disease. In normal breathing there is movement of the thorax and abdomen. Heavy, laboured breathing, confined chiefly to the abdominal wall with the thorax participating but little in the movements, signifies a painful condition of the chest, such as acute pleurisy and pneumonia. Exaggerated movements of the walls of the chest, on the other hand, are seen in disorders of the organs of the abdomen, such as in certain types of colic, peritonitis or other painful affections, when an attempt is made to limit the movements of the abdomen as much as possible.

Difficult or laboured breathing is known as dyspnoea and may occur when, for any reason, it is difficult for the animal to obtain the amount of oxygen it requires. This may be due to congestion or consolidation of the lungs as in pneumonia, to pleurisy, to tumours of the nose, to paralysis or swelling of the throat, foreign bodies and other causes. When chronic, it is seen in emphysema of the lungs ("broken-wind").

In severe dyspnoea, the horse stands with its front feet apart, the neck straight out, and the head extended upon the neck. The nostrils are widely dilated, the face has an anxious expression, the eyeballs protrude, there is mouth breathing and increased movements of the thoracic and abdominal walls. Grunting may be heard.

TENDONS—SPRAINED

THE FIBROUS structures situated below the knee and hock behind the cannon bones are often the seat of sprains, and are a very common cause of lameness in light horses.

Cause

Prolonged exertion, particularly at the gallop, and violent efforts or sudden jerks, especially in young or poorly conditioned animals, are common causes of sprain of the back tendons. Muscular fatigue plays an important part in sprain as this allows greater movement of joints, and stress of tendons and ligaments. This commonly occurs when a horse is forced to prolonged effort and becomes tired. Sprained tendons may also result from improper shoeing; allowing the toes of the feet to grow too long, as occurs when horses are allowed to wear their shoes for too long a period; poor conformation or over-training of young animals.

The flexor tendons, the suspensory ligament and the check ligament are more frequently involved than the extensor tendons. The tendons of the foreleg are more commonly affected than those of the hind. From an owner's point of view, the differential diagnosis between the various forms and situations of sprains is not important.

Symptoms

Heat, swelling, tenderness and lameness are the usual symptoms of sprained tendons. Other symptoms are: stumbling even when walking; digging the toe into the ground; knee and fetlock bent, with later thickening and "gumminess" of the leg. The degree of lameness varies according to the extent of the injury to the tendon fibres and the amount of haemorrhage and effusion. It is important to keep in mind that all heat and swelling in the region of the back tendons is not necessarily due to sprain of the tendons. Such a condition can be caused by an infection in the foot or mechanical injury to the part, such as a blow from the opposite foot.

Treatment

It is advisable to obtain the services of a veterinarian, at least for diagnosis and advice on the initial treatment of the sprained tendons. There are various methods of treatment, but the essential factor is rest. The shoes should be removed. Cold water applications from a hose have some merit when used sufficiently early, but treatment should include continued pressure on the tendons. The application of a pressure bandage straight away will probably give the best results. The object of the pressure is to promote reabsorption of the fluid which has formed in the tendon sheath, and to prevent further fluid forming. Special pads are available for binding evenly along the sides of the tendons. Alternatively, cotton wool or cotton wadding is placed evenly round the leg, care being taken to have it so thick that subsequent pressure of the bandage will not injure the skin. Over this is wound a long crepe bandage as tightly and as evenly as possible, so that it will exert even pressure over the whole of the injured surface and extend well above and below it. The padding should also project at each end to ensure that there is no cutting of the skin by the edges of the bandage. This pressure bandage should remain on for 24 hours. If it becomes loose, it should be removed, the leg massaged and the bandage re-applied. Such pressure should be maintained for at least a week, the bandage being removed night and morning, the leg rubbed, and the bandage re-applied.

In acute cases alternative methods of treatment are cold compresses, ice packs and evaporating lotions. Blistering may be carried out later if considered necessary, care being taken to place a ring of petroleum jelly around the top of the pastern, and in the heel to prevent the blister running. The horse should be tied up for 24 to 36 hours.

Early cases of sprained tendons may also be treated with kaolin and glycerine paste or the proprietary preparation, *Antiphlogistine*, spread on a piece of lint or cotton wool. The affected area should first be lightly coated with petroleum jelly or oil, and the dressing then applied reasonably hot and firmly bandaged to keep it in position. The dressing should be renewed every 24 hours.

Special shoeing, to raise the hind part of the foot and thus remove tension on the tendons, gives relief to the horse when sprain of certain tendons occurs.

A horse with a badly sprained tendon will be unfit for work for a month or six weeks, although he may appear to be sound before this time. Chronic sprained tendons are often incurable.

TETANUS

TETANUS, sometimes known as "lockjaw", is an acute infectious disease of all domestic animals and man. Horses, sheep and goats are particularly susceptible, but cattle, pigs, dogs and cats less so. The disease has a world-wide distribution, particularly in closely settled areas, and occurs mainly in horses as individual sporadic cases. The disease, which usually originates from infection of a wound, is characterized by spasms affecting the muscles of the face, neck, body and limbs, and all muscles supplied by the cerebro-spinal nerves. It is essentially an affliction of the nervous system and is not a blood infection.

Cause

The disease is caused by a toxin which is elaborated by the organism *Clostridium tetani*, when it gains entrance to deep punctured wounds, or any wound which seals over quickly and from which the air is excluded.

The tetanus germs form spores which are capable of living in the soil for long periods. When these spores gain entrance to a wound in which conditions are suitable for their propagation, they start to proliferate and at the same time produce a powerful toxin which affects the nervous system. Tetanus organisms occur quite commonly in the intestinal tract of animals without doing any harm, and are passed out in the droppings. This is the reason why infection is more likely to occur on heavily manured soils, or in horse yards, or wherever there is an accumulation of animal manure.

Predisposing Causes

When a horse develops tetanus, there is generally a history of injury. Wounds most prone to be infected are those which come in contact with the ground, or those which penetrate deeply into the tissues. Nails, splinters, stakes and other sharp objects are common causes. Infection may also occur from contaminated dust, which has blown on to a superficial wound, which scabs over quickly. Tetanus may also occur following fractures of bones, castration, tail docking, injuries to the mouth (sharp teeth) or injuries to the genital passages (from aid given in difficult foaling) and infection of the navel cord in foals.

Incubation Period

Although tetanus spores may lie dormant in the tissues for some months, and clinical symptoms of the disease may not be produced until the conditions are favourable for their propagation, it is common, if the germ has been introduced, for symptoms to develop after an incubation period which varies in different animals. In the horse it is between one and three weeks.

Symptoms

The main symptoms are stiffness of the muscles and tremors. The muscles of the neck and along the spine become involved, and the legs are moved in a stiff manner. The head is extended and the third eyelid (or haw) protrudes over the inner portion of the eye with a characteristic movement. This movement is very quick as the third eyelid moves out over the eye, but very slow on return. This occurs especially when the animal is disturbed. Noise or disturbance throws the animal into increased spasms of the affected muscles. The tail

223

is usually slightly elevated and stiff and the ears are erect. The jaws become set (locked), the animal is unable to eat and saliva may drool from the mouth. As the disease progresses, the horse adopts a characteristic attitude with fore and hind legs extended (saw-horse stance). Breathing becomes difficult, the lips are drawn tightly over the teeth, the nostrils are dilated and the animal, which has an anxious expression, may sweat profusely. Constipation sets in early in the attack. Temperature is not much changed at first, but may rise to 108° F. just before death. In severe attacks, recovery seldom occurs and death takes place in three to five days or a little longer. The mortality rate is about 80 per cent.

Those cases that set in slowly after a long incubation period, and in which the symptoms are not severe, may recover if carefully nursed in proper surroundings. A convalescent period of several months is required before the horse is worked again.

Tetanus may possibly be confounded with other disease conditions, such as strychnine poisoning, spinal meningitis and forage poisoning. The typical muscular spasms of tetanus, the movement of the third eyelid across the eye, coupled with the possible history of a wound, should assist in diagnosis.

Treatment

If the horse is a valuable animal, or if for sentimental reasons it is desired to do everything possible to save the animal, a veterinary surgeon should be called in. He will treat the animal with large doses of tetanus antitoxin and will administer antibiotic drugs and muscle-relaxing agents. The treatment is costly and the results uncertain. Destruction of the horse might be the most humane action.

As already pointed out, mild cases of tetanus may recover with good nursing. The horse should be kept quiet in a darkened, roomy stall, away from other animals, the floor being bedded with sawdust, sand or short straw. A fresh supply of cool drinking water should be placed in a convenient position on a level with the horse's head. Soft, sloppy, easily-digested foods should be freshly prepared, and placed at head level. The horse can often suck up liquids such as thin oatmeal gruel prepared with milk, even though the jaws are "locked". It is very important to keep up the animal's strength and, if it can masticate at all, freshly prepared bran mashes, chopped greenstuff or even a little good quality cereal chaff and crushed oats will tempt the horse to eat.

If the animal will take Epsom salts or potassium nitrate (nitre) in the feed, these may be given in small quantities or dissolved in the drinking water. Drenching should not be attempted, and even the use of a stomach tube is undesirable, as attempts to pass the tube tend to throw the horse into a spasm. Under certain circumstances, it may be necessary to sling the horse. Additional supportive treatment, including intravenous feeding, would be given by a veterinarian.

If the wound can be located, it should be cleansed with hydrogen peroxide, a strong solution of *Condy's* crystals, or a 4 per cent carbolic acid solution. A punctured wound in the foot must be pared out, antiseptics applied, and then packed with antibiotic ointment. Frequent irrigation of a wound is inadvisable as this may facilitate absorption of the toxin.

During nursing of the animal, the attendant must move quietly and be careful to prevent unnecessary excitement, which might increase the spasms.

Prevention

When a horse has sustained a severe or punctured wound, arrangements should be made for a veterinary surgeon to administer tetanus antitoxin, which is of far greater value as a preventive than as a curative agent. The preventive action lasts only for ten to fourteen days which is, however, usually sufficient to prevent the disease developing.

As a routine procedure, tetanus toxoid is used to immunize animals against the disease, and horse-owners are advised to give serious consideration to having their horses protected against tetanus in this manner. Immunity is conferred in approximately two weeks after the initial injections, given at intervals of a month, when the horse will be immune to tetanus for at least a year. If annual "booster" injections are given, horses will remain immune from tetanus.

THOROUGHPIN

THIS unusual term is applied to a chronic synovitis (or inflammation of the synovial sheath) of the deep flexor tendon at the back of the hock, and distension of the membrane by fluid. It should be differentiated from bog spavin which is a chronic synovitis of the hock joint with distension of the joint capsule. In thoroughpin, the swelling is seen on either side of the hock in front of the hamstring about the level of the "point of the hock". It varies in size and may be more noticeable on the inside or on the outside. Pressure with the fingers on the swelling at one side of the leg causes a corresponding or even greater filling on the opposite side.

Cause

A thoroughpin usually results from excessive strain on the flexor tendon as it passes around the hock. This results in inflammation and

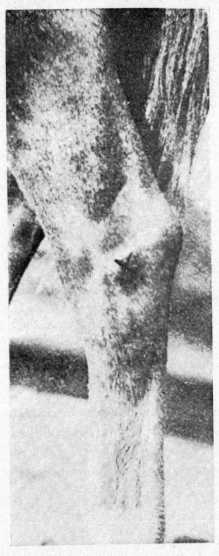

Fig. 83 Thoroughpin at X.
(United States Department of Agriculture)

"filling" of the tendon sheath. The condition was formerly more commonly seen in draught horses, when it was associated with excessive exertion when backing heavy loads, especially on a slippery surface. It is also seen in light horses, in which the condition may result from jumping, pulling up suddenly when galloping, and from other forms of sudden strain on the tendons such as kicks and other injuries. On the other hand, thoroughpin is seen in horses in which there is no history of excessive strain and, as in the case of bog spavin, may be associated with defective conformation. The condition is sometimes seen in young horses, and may disappear spontaneously.

Symptoms .

Slight lameness may be evident when the condition first occurs, but this is not severe unless the flexor tendon has been severely sprained. After the lesion becomes chronic, it causes no inconvenience to the horse and does not interfere with its work. The blemish is, of course, unsightly and depreciates the value of the animal.

Treatment

In those cases which arise gradually, without causing any inconvenience, and where the swelling is often quite small, no treatment is warranted. The swelling may slowly increase in size or it may diminish and, especially in the case of young horses, disappear. For acute cases which have followed sprain of the flexor tendon, cold water applications with a hose are beneficial in reducing inflammation. Cooling astringent lotions may also be used. A pressure bandage with cotton wool, as recommended for the treatment of bog spavin, is useful in reducing the swelling if it can be well applied. Rest is, of course, essential. Any break in the skin must be treated as an open wound.

If the condition becomes chronic, it is doubtful if any treatment will be entirely successful, but as the usefulness of the horse is not impaired by the swelling, the only disadvantage is the blemish.

Aspiration of the fluid and corticosteroid injections by a veterinarian, if carried out early, may bring about lasting reduction of the swelling.

THRUSH

IN HORSES the term "thrush" is applied to a disease affecting the cleft of the frog in which there is a degenerative condition of the horn, characterized by a black and offensive discharge from the cleft.

Q

Cause

The condition results from a bacterial infection and catarrhal inflammation of the glands deep in the cleft of the frog.

The frog is normally resistant to bacterial invasion, but may deteriorate and become susceptible as the result of long-continued exposure to excessively wet or filthy stable floors and yards.

Thrush can also occur under dry conditions in horses with contracted feet and where there is little or no frog pressure.

Symptoms

Attention is usually drawn first to the condition of thrush by the characteristic foul smell of the discharge from the affected frog. The frog may be wasted and fissured, and the horn soft and easily detachable in the depth of the cleft. Mild thrush rarely causes lameness. In more advanced cases of the disease, the sensitive structures become involved, the frog is hot and tender to pressure, and there may be tenderness of the heels and coronet. Under such circumstances, lameness occurs.

Treatment

Attention to stable hygiene and cleanliness of the foot is, of course, essential. When the condition has arisen as the result of lack of frog pressure, this should be rectified. Remove the shoes and rasp down the heels and walls as low as possible, without making the foot tender, the object being to obtain frog pressure as soon as possible. Good frog pressure is essential for a healthy foot.

As far as the actual treatment of lesions is concerned, the first step is to clean out the cleft of the frog with a stiff brush and warm soap and water and then to trim away any loose pieces of the frog. Subsequent treatment will depend on the seriousness of the condition. Poulticing may be of value at this stage, followed by the application of some suitable astringent antiseptic dressing, such as 1 oz. of sulphate of zinc and 1 oz. of lead acetate in a pint of water, to be well shaken before application. A five per cent solution of bluestone (1 oz. bluestone to a pint of water) is also useful. These dressings have both antiseptic and hardening properties. Many others have a similar value.

It may be necessary to syringe out a suppurating area with a non-irritant antiseptic solution, such as five per cent *Dettol* (2 tablespoonfuls to a pint of water) or *Cetavlon*, at least once a day. Sulphonamide and antibiotic powders can also be used to advantage, and a dry dressing of calomel dusted on once or twice a day is also effective, especially in early cases.

228

If the horse can be turned out into a grass paddock, it will obtain the necessary exercise, otherwise it should be exercised several times a day on soft dry ground.

With restoration, as far as possible, of frog pressure, and with general cleanliness and careful dressing, a cure is nearly always obtained.

TONGUE—INFLAMMATION OF

APART from actinomycosis or actinobacillosis and "cancer" of the tongue of the horse, which occur rarely, inflammation of the tongue, which is called glossitis, not uncommonly occurs.

Causes

The common causes of inflammation and injury to the tongue are penetration by grass seeds, irregularities of the teeth, bit injuries, or putting a twitch on the tongue (which should never be done).

Symptoms

Swelling and protrusion of the tongue, difficulty in mastication and swallowing and dribbling of saliva.

The sides and underneath of the tongue should be examined for grass seeds or wounds, and the top of the tongue for bit injuries. The teeth should also be checked for sharp projections and other irregularities.

Treatment

Bathe the affected area with a saturated solution of boracic acid or chlorate of potash ($\frac{1}{2}$ oz. to a pint of water). These drugs may also be mixed with honey and used as an electuary applied with a smooth flat stick to the tongue. Wounds of the tongue usually heal well.

Feed the horse on soft foods, such as bran mashes and gruels, and cut green feed.

TUBERCULOSIS

ALTHOUGH tuberculosis is a common disease in cattle, pigs and poultry, it occurs only rarely in the horse. When it does occur, it is usually in the abdominal form, caused by the bovine type of organism. It is sometimes contracted by foals which are given milk from a tubercular cow.

In the horse, the disease is usually of a chronic character and is often not suspected until it is fairly well advanced.

The organs most commonly affected are the mesenteric lymph glands, the intestines and spleen. Lesions are also seen in the bones, including the neck bones, less commonly in the lungs and elsewhere in the body. The symptoms vary according to the location of the disease. Common symptoms are unthriftiness, loss of condition, capricious appetite, associated sometimes with coughing and nasal discharges when there are pulmonary lesions.

When the neck bones of the horse are affected, an osteomyelitis develops, which causes stiffness of the neck.

The disease may be diagnosed by a tuberculin test, of which the subcutaneous tuberculin test seems to be the most reliable.

Treatment of the disease in the horse, as with other animals, is not practicable.

TUMOURS

PRACTICALLY all the tissues and organs of the body are susceptible to the formation of tumours, which may be benign or malignant.

The term "cancer" is popularly applied to malignant tumours or neoplasms, characterized by the fact that they are usually non-capsulated and invade surrounding tissues of the part in which they develop; they grow rapidly and have a marked influence on the general health of the animal. Furthermore, there is a tendency for them to recur after an operation for removal. This results from a continued growth of particles which escape removal, or of particles which have spread before the operation to other parts and organs, through the medium of the blood circulation or by the lymphatic system.

On the other hand, benign tumours are generally well encapsulated and do not infiltrate the surrounding tissues. They grow slowly and, depending on their situation, seldom disturb the general health. They are less likely to recur if surgically removed and do not produce secondary growths in other parts of the body.

Two neoplasms are found fairly commonly in horses. Cancer of the eye, which occurs on the third eyelid, the cornea or the upper or lower eyelid, spreads rapidly, and involves the whole eye and surrounding structures.

This condition is amenable to operation in the early stages, especially if the growth commences on the third eyelid. The whole eyelid, together with the growth, is removed. Care should be taken not to mistake the early stage of the growth with *habronemic granuloma* (see *Eye—Habronemic Conjunctivitis*).

Melanotic tumour, or melanosis, is a malignant growth which occurs especially in aged grey horses. This dark-coloured tumour, which may appear in various parts of the body, occurs commonly at the root of the tail and about the anus, sheath and crest. (See *Melanoma*)

With few exceptions, as in the case of certain benign tumours, well-performed surgery is the only satisfactory treatment for tumours in the horse. Although this might be quite satisfactory in certain cases such as an early eye "cancer", it is seldom satisfactory in the case of melanosis in the horse.

TWISTED BOWEL

UNDER this heading is included also strangulation and intussusception—telescoping—of the bowel. All these conditions are very serious, and lead to intestinal obstruction, which generally terminates in death of the animal.

A twisting of the bowel upon itself is referred to as a volvulus. It is most likely to occur during strenuous exercise, such as violent rolling, jumping, or other sudden bodily movements, or be associated with a severe attack of colic.

Intestinal strangulation is seen in cases of inguinal or umbilical hernia, or may result from a twist of the bowel. Long-necked tumours in the mesentery sometimes become twisted around a part of the small intestine and cause strangulation.

Intussusception of the bowel is a slipping or telescoping of a portion of the intestine into another portion immediately adjoining, like a partially turned-in glove finger. This may occur at any part of the bowels, but is more frequent in the small intestines. The telescoped portion may be small—two or three inches only—or extensive, measuring several feet. The causes include irregular or excessive peristaltic movements, as may result from profuse diarrhoea, inflammation of the bowels and worm infection. Foals are most commonly affected by this condition.

Symptoms

The symptoms of all the above conditions are similar, and a non-professional person is unlikely to be able to make a definite diagnosis. There is a sudden onset of acute colicky pain. The horse rolls, paws the ground, breaks out in a sweat, and shows increased respiration and heart rate. The mucous membranes of the eyes and nose are usually congested. A little dung may be passed at first, followed by constipation. Severe straining occurs in some cases of intussusception and this may be regarded with suspicion when it occurs. As death approaches, the horse sweats profusely, presents an anxious countenance, the legs and ears become cold, and there is often freedom from pain just before death. Most cases end fatally within twelve to twenty-four hours.

Treatment

There should be no delay in obtaining the services of a veterinarian. Surgery may save the life of the patient. An ounce of chloral hydrate in a pint of thin gruel may be given to relieve the pain.

UDDER—INFLAMMATION OF

See *Mastitis*

ULCER

Black's Veterinary Dictionary defines an ulcer as, "a breach on the surface of the skin, or on the surface of any mucous or other membrane of a cavity of the body, which does not tend to heal". It is a process of destruction involving the death of small portions of healthy tissue around the edge, which causes the ulcer to spread. This is called ulceration.

There are various types of ulcers, and specific ulcers occur in association with a number of diseases.

Spontaneous or primary ulcers, such as those that follow injury anywhere on the surface of the skin, in the mouth and on the tongue, are due to a continuous irritant on the wound, which prevents healing.

Such irritation may be caused by bacteria, the use of strong antiseptics, constant rubbing of the wound by harness or, in the case of the mouth, by the irritating influence of infected, loose or irregular teeth on the cheek or tongue. Debility and disturbances of circulation are predisposing causes.

Treatment

Specific ulcers associated with various diseases usually heal under general treatment or when the disease has run its course.

In the case of spontaneous ulcers, the first thing is to remove the exciting cause. The ulcer should be cleaned up with some weak antiseptic solution and any pieces of dead tissue on the surface removed. It may now be treated with a stimulating healing lotion, such as *white lotion* (1 oz. lead acetate, 1 oz. zinc sulphate, 1 pint of water), or dusted with sulphonamide or antibiotic powders. The horse should be rested, preferably in a well-grassed paddock, kept under observation and treated as required.

A seriously-inflamed or chronic ulcer requires professional attention.

232

URINARY CALCULI—("STONE" OR "GRAVEL") (Urolithiasis)

THE HORSE is not uncommonly affected by urinary calculi, either in the kidneys, ureters (tubes leading from kidneys to the bladder), bladder, or urethra. These calculi or "stones", as they are commonly called, are formed from various salts normally excreted in the urine. The more common calculi found in the horse consist of calcium carbonate, calcium phosphate and magnesium carbonate.

Although calculi may occur anywhere along the urinary tract, they are most commonly found in the bladder of the horse. Here they occur as egg-shaped or flat, hard, yellowish grey concretions, the surfaces of which are either smooth or mulberry-like, and they vary in size from a small stone up to a concretion the size of a man's fist. In addition to these stone-like concretions, there may also be present a "gravel" or sand-like sediment commonly referred to as "urinary gravel" or "urinary sand".

Several small calculi or one large calculus may sometimes occur in the pelvis of the kidney, and be undiagnosed until death of the animal, when they are seen at post-mortem examination.

Those calculi which are found in the passages leading from the kidney to the bladder are simply small renal calculi that have escaped from the pelvis of the kidney. If they completely block the ureter, the retained urine causes destructive pressure in the kidney.

Urethral calculi are less frequent in horses than in sheep and cattle because of the larger size of the urethra in the horse, and the absence of the S-shaped curve which occurs in the penis of the former animals. The calculi which are arrested in the urethra are not formed there, but consist of cystic calculi which have been small enough to pass through the neck of the bladder, but which are too large to pass through the whole length of the urethra (in the male) and so escape. This trouble is most unlikely to occur in the mare.

Still other calculi occur in the horse, namely concretions in the sheath, and these are known as preputial calculi. Within the sheath, the concretions are usually of soft, cheese-like sebaceous matter and not true calculi, but the latter do occur. Both may interfere with the flow of urine, but are easily removed by the fingers.

Cause

The underlying causes of urinary calculi (or urolithiasis) are not fully understood and are still the subject of scientific investigation. Without going into a lot of detail as to how calculi in the urinary tract of the horse might be formed, it can be said that the calculi occur under varied conditions and it seems unlikely that there is a common factor in the causation of the different types of calculi.

Symptoms

Generally, the symptoms of urinary calculi are those of colicky pain, appearing suddenly, very often following exhausting work; straining and repeated efforts to urinate; interruption in the flow of urine; presence of blood in the urine; presence of sand-like deposit in the urine; stiffness of gait of the hind legs and movement of the tail.

In the case of "stone" in the bladder, the rough mulberry-like calculi, especially, lead to irritation and wounding of the mucous membrane of the bladder with bleeding. This occurs most commonly when the horse is ridden or driven. When the horse is pulled up and proceeds to urinate, there follows the passage of blood stained urine.

The presence of the stone or stones in the bladder can be readily ascertained by placing the hand and arm into the rectum and feeling down on to the bladder.

Treatment

It will be appreciated that the treatment for obstructive calculi in various positions in the urinary tract is difficult, and is usually a case for surgery by an experienced veterinarian. It is not practicable to dissolve the calculi by medical means, but veterinarians have at their disposal certain drugs which may prevent increase in the size of existing calculi and the development of new ones. Drugs are also available to relax the urethral muscle and allow the obstructing "stone" to pass on, but success depends on very early treatment.

The removal of a large stone in the bladder, whilst presenting great difficulties and the necessity for a major operation under a general anaesthetic in the case of a stallion or gelding, can, in the case of a mare, be comparatively easily carried out through the short female urethra which is only two to three inches in length. The female urethra opens on to the floor of the vagina about four inches from the outside. It is possible for a veterinarian, with his hand in the vagina, to remove the stone by hand through the urethra, which is capable of remarkable dilation if sufficient care and patience are exercised in the process. Special forceps greatly facilitate the work.

URINE SUPPRESSION AND URINE RETENTION

See *Suppression of Urine*

URTICARIA
See *Nettle Rash*

UTERUS—DISEASES OF
See *Metritis*

VAGINITIS (Inflammation of the Vagina)

VAGINITIS may exist independently, but it is more commonly associated with metritis (inflammation of the womb) or cervicitis (inflammation of the neck of the womb).

Cause

Generally due to specific infections; commonly follows difficult parturition which requires manual assistance and the use of instruments or ropes to remove the foal; may be caused by any situation leading to irritation, bruising or wounding of the mucous membrane of the vagina, with or without secondary infection. It sometimes follows retention of the afterbirth and may mask the more serious condition of metritis.

Infections of the vagina can play a part in preventing conception.

Symptoms

The lips of the vulva and the lining membrane of the vagina are more or less swollen and the latter is congested and often a bright red colour. Sometimes there are small, pearl-like or warty lumps or outgrowths on the floor of the vagina. The mare switches the tail and exhibits signs similar to "horsing" with dribbling of urine. After the inflammation has existed for several days, a discharge appears, which is at first clear and sometimes streaked with blood, but which later becomes thicker, with pus and mucus. This usually causes soiling of the tail, thighs and hocks. The temperature may be raised.

Treatment

As a rule, simple vaginitis is not very serious. The inflammation often subsides in the course of a few days, or rapidly yields to treatment. If left untreated it may become chronic. Although this may not affect the general health of the mare, it may result in failure of the mare to get in foal.

Antibiotic and other antiseptic powders in "puffer packs" might be used in the treatment of simple vaginitis, but because of the common association of vaginitis with metritis and cervicitis, the services of a veterinarian should be obtained in order that a thorough examination of the mare can be carried out for evidence of these conditions.

(See also *Metritis*)

WARTS (Equine Cutaneous Papillomatosis)

WARTS, or cutaneous papillomas as they are technically called, are solid outgrowths of epidermis, which appear as small elevated horny masses, usually on the muzzle, nose, and lips. They seldom occur elsewhere on the body. They may remain flat and small, but some increase greatly in size or become pendulous. They are more common in young horses and may be few in number or quite numerous.

When not complicated by other conditions, warts are non-inflammatory and painless and usually cause little inconvenience. Around the mouth they may interfere with feeding and, when occurring around the nostrils, they may obstruct breathing.

Warts usually disappear spontaneously after a few months but may persist for six months and sometimes longer, when they can be responsible for loss of condition.

Cause

The disease is caused by a virus, and is infectious. The disease has been transmitted experimentally to young horses by injection, or by application of a suspension of wart tissue to scarified skin. Under natural conditions, transmission of the disease is believed to take place by direct contact with infected horses through a break in the skin, or when animals with an abrasion of the skin rub against rails, posts or other objects which have become contaminated with the virus. Halters, headstalls and grooming equipment can spread the disease.

Although the virus is relatively resistant, it is not known how long it will remain alive on inanimate objects.

Treatment

As already indicated, the disease is self-limiting and eventually disappears. After recovery, the horse is immune to further infection. Vaccines are used, both for the treatment and prevention of the disease, but, unless the vaccine is prepared from the virus of equine cutaneous papillomatosis, it is likely to be ineffective. Vaccines prepared from wart tissue of the affected animal give better results.

Other treatments include the injection of proprietary preparations containing antimony and bismuth, local application of glacial acetic acid or of a caustic potash stick. When the latter two are used, care should be taken that only the warts are treated, and that the skin around them is protected with petroleum jelly. Several applications will be necessary, at intervals of a few days.

The tendency for spontaneous recovery to occur makes assessment of the results of treatment difficult.

Warts may also be removed surgically, but the operation should not be carried out in the early stage of development, as this will often stimulate the growth of remaining warts and cause others to appear. Pendulous warts, which are not common in horses, may sometimes be successfully removed by ligation with a strong thread close to the base.

Bearing in mind that the disease is infectious, efforts should be made to keep affected horses apart from healthy animals.

WATERING

A HORSE requires a daily average of about 8 gallons of water. In very hot weather it will drink up to 15 gallons. The quantity varies not only with the weather and the amount of work performed, but also with the character of the feed. Stabled horses should be watered at least three times a day before feeding, and paddocked horses should have an ample supply of good clean water available to them at all times.

Water obtained from pools or shallow wells contaminated with surface drainage or decomposing organic matter frequently leads to digestive upsets, while water containing a large amount of sediment causes mechanical irritation of the mucous membrane of the stomach and intestines and may cause the condition known as sand colic.

A horse may be permitted to drink when hot if the quantity allowed is not too great. After prolonged exertion or fast work, the body fluids are depleted. The animal will not eat sufficiently until its thirst has at least been partially satisfied. Water should be given first, and while the animal is still warm is the best time to give it. However, after hard or fast work, drinking should not be permitted until the breathing has returned to normal. It is preferable to provide small quantities at intervals than to allow unlimited water, particularly if the water is very cold. Small quantities of water can be given if desired an hour after the completion of feeding.

After a long trek, it is a good plan to water a mile or so before the journey's end and take the horse in slowly afterwards. This prevents chills and colic due to the ingestion of a large quantity of water when in an exhausted state.

Girths should always be loosened before watering, and horses allowed ample time to drink. They should not be led away the first time they raise their heads from the water.

WEAVING

WEAVING is a vice or nervous habit acquired by many wild animals in captivity and sometimes by horses, especially those that are stabled for long periods. The animal rocks itself to and fro continually, swinging the head and neck and front part of the body, sometimes lifting each fore foot in turn as the body is swayed to the opposite side. Some horses practise the vice occasionally, while others do it constantly. A constant weaver wears itself out to the extent that its working capacity is affected.

Idleness and boredom appear to predispose to weaving and, as with other vices, the habit is likely to be copied by other horses in a stable. It is advisable, therefore, to keep a weaver away from other horses, so that they will not be disturbed and learn the trick from observation. It has been suggested that an uneven stable floor will start a horse weaving.

Once acquired, the habit of weaving is difficult to break. Various devices are adopted to control the weaving, but the confirmed weaver usually overcomes these and continues to weave even if in a restricted manner. A simple method of controlling weaving is to tie the horse to side rings. The horse should be given plenty of exercise or regular work and be turned out into a grass paddock, rather than being stabled. If the horse has to be stabled, care should be taken that the stable floor is even, and plenty of good bedding should be provided to encourage the horse to lie down.

WEED

THIS unscientific term, when applied to the horse, means sporadic lymphangitis ("Monday morning disease" or "Big-leg").

See *Lymphangitis (Sporadic)*

WEIGHTS AND MEASURES

THE following are the weights and measures most likely to be used by horse owners. The relationship between the British System and the Metric System is also given.

WEIGHTS

BRITISH SYSTEM

Apothecaries'
(Used when dealing with drugs)

60 grains	=	1 dram
8 drams	=	1 ounce (480 grains)
12 ounces	=	1 pound

238

Avoirdupois

(Used when weighing foodstuffs, materials for licks, and also in the
preparation of foot-rot bath solutions and so on)

16	ounces	= 1 pound
14	pounds	= 1 stone
2	stones	= 1 quarter
4	quarters	= 1 hundredweight
20	hundredweight	= 1 ton
1	ounce (avoirdupois)	= 437½ grains (apothecaries)

METRIC SYSTEM

The chief unit of weight or measure of mass is the gramme (g.).

1 kilogramme	=	1000 grammes
1 hectogramme	=	100 grammes
1 decagramme	=	10 grammes
1 gramme	=	weight of 1 cubic centimetre of water
1 decigramme	=	tenth part of 1 gramme or 0·1 gramme
1 centigramme	=	hundredth part of 1 gramme or 0·01 gramme
1 milligramme	=	thousandth part of 1 gramme or 0·001 gramme

Conversion

1 ounce (avoirdupois) = 437½ grains = 28·35 grammes
(usually taken as 30 grammes)

1 pound (avoirdupois) = 16 oz. = 7000 grains
= 453·6 grammes

1 gramme = 15 grains (approx.)

1 scruple = 20 grains

CAPACITY

BRITISH SYSTEM

For liquids the measure used is as follows:

60	minims (drops)	= 1 fluid dram
8	fluid drams	= 1 fluid ounce
20	fluid ounces (or 4 gills)	= 1 pint
2	pints	= 1 quart
8	pints (4 quarts)	= 1 gallon = 10 pounds (water)

The unit of capacity in the Metric system is the litre.

1 millilitre	=	1 cubic centimetre
10 millilitres	=	1 centilitre
10 centilitres	=	1 decilitre
10 decilitres	=	1 litre

Conversion

1 cubic centimetre (c.c.) or 1 millilitre (ml.) of water weighs 1 gramme and equals 17 minims (approx.). (It will be seen that a cubic centimetre is the same as a millilitre—the latter term being now commonly used.)

30 cubic centimetres or millilitres	= 1 fluid ounce
1000 cubic centimetres or millilitres	= 1 litre = 1·75 pints

LENGTH

1 metre (m.)	= 100 centimetres (cm.) = 1000 millimetres (mm.) = 39·37 inches
1 kilometre (km.)	= 1000 metres = $\frac{5}{8}$ mile (approx.)
1 inch	= 25·4 millimetres
1 mile	= 1760 yards = 5280 feet
	= 1·6 kilometres (approx.)

HOUSEHOLD MEASURES

DOMESTIC measures cannot be relied upon, as cups, spoons and glasses vary in size. A proper graduated measuring glass, which costs only a few cents, should be kept on hand for measuring liquids, and good scales and proper weights used for solids. Sometimes, however, these are not available when required and the following rough equivalents may be used for fluids.

Stamped quart bottle	= 40 fluid oz. (to line, or shoulder)
Wine bottle	= 26 fluid oz. (approximately)
Common tumblers	= 8-10 fluid oz.
Breakfast cup	= 8-10 fluid oz.
Teacup	= 5-7 fluid oz.
Egg cup	= 1¼-1½ fluid oz.
Tablespoon	= ½-1 fluid oz.
Dessertspoon	= 2-3 fluid drams
Teaspoon (average)	= 1 fluid dram (60 minims)
1 drop	= 1 minim

The foregoing measures apply only to watery liquids; solids, of course, vary so greatly in weight that they cannot be estimated in this way.

A stamped grocery or other empty carton or tin should never be used to measure by weight an equal quantity of another solid.

PERCENTAGE SOLUTIONS

THE mixing of antiseptic washes or other solutions is often a matter of difficulty when the only directions given are to use a certain percentage solution. The percentage solutions most commonly used in veterinary work for horses are 1, 2, 5 and 10 per cent.

For all practical purposes these may be prepared as follows:

Percentage

1 = 100 minims or approximately 1½ teaspoonfuls to 1 pint of water.

2 = 200 minims or approximately 3 teaspoonfuls to 1 pint of water.

5 = 1 fluid oz. and 20 minims or approximately 2 tablespoonfuls to 1 pint of water.

10 = 2 fluid oz. and 40 minims or approximately 4 tablespoonfuls to 1 pint of water.

The following measurements may also be of use:

Percentage

½ = 1 fluid oz. in 10 pints (Imp.) or 1¼ gallons.

1 = 1 fluid oz. in 5 pints (Imp.) or 2½ quarts.

5 = 1 fluid oz. in 1 pint (Imp.).

10 = 2 fluid oz. in 1 pint (Imp.).

It sometimes happens that the horse-owner is told to make percentage solutions of solids in liquids. This is more difficult and necessitates the use of scales to weigh the solids.

To make a 1 per cent solution of a solid in a liquid take 4½ grains of the solid to 1 oz. of liquid or 90 grains to 1 pint of liquid (approximately 1½ oz. to a gallon).

To make a 2 per cent solution take 9 grains to the ounce or 180 grains (3 drams) to the pint (approximately 3 oz. to 1 gallon).

To make a 5 per cent solution take 22 grains to the ounce or 1 oz. to the pint (½ lb. to 1 gallon).

To make a 10 per cent solution take 44 grains to the ounce or 2 oz. to the pint (1 lb. to 1 gallon).

These equivalents are only approximate but close enough for general purposes.

WHISTLING
See *Roaring and Whistling*

WHEAT—ENGORGEMENT WITH
See *Colic*

WIND—BROKEN
See *Broken-Wind*

WINDGALLS
A WINDGALL is defined as a soft fluid-filled tumour or swelling in the region of the fetlock joint of the horse. The common types of windgalls recognized are articular windgall, in which the bursa of the fetlock joint is involved, and tendinous windgall, when the swelling occurs in the tendon sheath surrounding the flexor tendon at the back of the leg. Independent bursae also develop between bone and tendon. Windgalls appear in the form of soft puffy swellings, varying in size from a pea to a walnut or larger. They occur at the back of the fetlock joint and are most commonly seen in the foreleg.

Cause

Windgalls occur as the result of sudden or sustained strain thrown upon the fetlock joint or the tendons at the back of the leg with resultant inflammation of the bursa of the joint or the tendon sheath. They occur in young animals that are put to work too soon, and are quite common in old horses. They are not uncommonly seen in trotters and jumpers. Faulty conformation, such as short pasterns and upright shoulders, are contributing causes.

Symptoms

Usually windgalls are painless and only cause lameness under certain conditions. Lameness occurs during the early stages of inflammation, or when the tumour is large and situated to the inside of the leg and is injured by interference, causing further inflammation of the sac and stumbling. In long-standing cases, the tumours are hardened, the walls being converted into fibrous tissue or even ossified (becoming bone-like)

242

Treatment

As windgalls are of little consequence except for being unsightly, and rarely cause lameness, treatment is not very important. When the condition occurs in young animals, it frequently clears up without treatment as the animal grows older. On the other hand, windgalls do become well established and such chronic cases are difficult to clear up. Treatment at this stage is usually only temporarily successful, the dilation returning when the animal is returned to work.

When in the acute stage, it is useful to apply hot fomentations followed by the application of a cold water bandage or cold water irrigation by means of a hose. Massage, and bandaging with evenly-distributed pressure, will also be found advantageous in reducing the swelling. Rest is an important part of treatment and the horse should be spelled and brought into work again gradually. Should inflammation persist and the animal be lame, excess fluid can be withdrawn and corticosteroid injections given by a veterinary surgeon. In more chronic cases, blistering and firing are sometimes carried out by veterinarians.

WIND-SUCKING
See *Crib-biting and Wind-sucking*

WITHERS, FISTULOUS
See *Fistulous Withers* and *Poll Evil*

WOMB—INFLAMMATION OF
See *Metritis*

WORMS
See *Parasites—Internal*

WOUNDS
OF ALL domestic animals, the horse is probably the most subject to accidental wounds. Horse-owners, particularly in the country, are often called upon to use their own ingenuity in treating animals which have been injured from a variety of causes. In this connection, the owner frequently places great reliance on the value of some particular ointment or dressing with which he is familiar. Not only are these dressings of very little benefit in the healing of wounds but they frequently retard the healing processes.

R

In the usual rural environment in Australia, two factors favour the healing of wounds in stock (1) the relatively large area over which the animal may roam with low risk of exposure to heavily-contaminated areas, and (2) the clear dry climate which keeps the surface of the wound dry, which is very important. The free movement of the animal also mechanically brings about natural drainage of the wound, and drainage is perhaps the most important factor in wound treatment.

The treatment of wounds of animals confined to stables and stalls is fraught with far greater risks.

Classification of Wounds

For convenience, wounds may be classified under five main headings:

1. Simple incised wounds—clean cut edges.
2. Abrasions—surface layers of skin destroyed by friction.
3. Lacerated wounds—torn edges; portions of skin, muscle and other tissue torn away.
4. Punctured wounds—deep penetration by pointed slender objects, frequent in horse's feet, such as nail pricks, and always dangerous because of the possibility of tetanus and other germ infection.
5. Contused wounds or bruises—diffuse damage about actual wound, blood and lymph invading neighbouring parts.

Healing Processes

There are four processes of healing; (1) healing by first intention; (2) healing by granulation; (3) healing under a scab; (4) union of granulating surfaces.

Healing by first intention is the immediate healing of two clean cut surfaces without complication. In large animals, other than in the case of surgical wounds, this seldom occurs. Most wounds in large animals can be looked upon as infected or septic, that is contamination of the wound by germs has taken place. This may not be serious, and is commonly controlled by natural processes.

Healing by granulation is the most common way by which wound repair in the horse takes place. Granulation tissue is newly-developed tissue composed of minute blood-vessels and cells producing fibrous tissue. This may be seen initially as tiny greyish-white flecks which appear over the surface of the wound. These spots gradually extend to cover the surface of the exposed area. This new tissue is richly supplied with blood vessels, and bleeds freely if damaged. The granulation tissue then grows together, filling up the gap in the wounded area. The wound is now impervious to bacterial invasion and infection is prevented. Healing proceeds by an outgrowth of skin cells which gradually cover the area. If, however, the surface of the wound is interfered with by rubbing, irritant dressings or other over-zealous treatment, excessive granulation tissue is formed, growing freely above the surface. This is the so-called "proud flesh", which can also occur under other unfavourable conditions.

Healing under a scab is granulation going on under a protective covering of coagulated lymph and white cells. It occurs in surface wounds and is a normal process of repair.

Union of granulating surfaces explains itself; when the granulations meet they unite to form a continuous layer.

Treatment of Wounds

Serious wounds call for the services of a veterinarian. There may be severe bleeding which, although temporarily arrested by pressure packs or a tourniquet, must be permanently stopped by tying-off the blood vessels. Deep punctured wounds, in addition to local treatment, will call for the injection of tetanus antitoxin and an antibiotic.

In various types of wounds, haemorrhage is likely to occur from the cutting of arteries or veins, the former being the more serious. Bleeding from an artery can be recognized by the manner in which the blood spurts in jets. The blood is also of a brighter red colour than that from the veins. When veins only are cut, the blood pours out in a continuous stream. Bleeding must be arrested before any attempt is made to dress the wound.

The loss of one or two quarts of blood by a robust horse is not dangerous, but if bleeding is long continued, severe weakening, and eventually death, will result. Whilst awaiting the arrival of the veterinarian, it may be possible to stop the flow of blood, at least temporarily, by the application of pressure over the part with a pad of sterile gauze, or clean cloth preferably sterilized by boiling. Direct pressure on the wound for five or ten minutes will allow clotting to occur. Should this not be effective and the wound be in a position where a bandage can be applied, a sterile pad may be bandaged over the wound. If this is not possible, pack the wound with sterile gauze or cotton wool and insert one or two large safety-pins through the skin of the wound to hold in the gauze, and then wind some fine string around the safety-pins in a figure-of-eight fashion to exert pressure. This should be removed carefully in 12 to 24 hours if professional assistance has not been available. If the wound is on a limb and the pressure bandage is not holding the bleeding, a tourniquet may be applied and adjusted above the injury. This may be done by applying a thick, twisted cloth about the leg and tying it loosely. A stick is then inserted in the space between the cloth and the leg and twisted to a degree of tightness only sufficient to stop the bleeding. On no account should the tourniquet be applied too tightly, and it should be loosened every twenty minutes so that the blood flow beyond the wound is not cut off entirely. The use of a tourniquet should be avoided if possible, as in unskilled hands it frequently leads to damage to the skin and tissue.

No substance, for example flour or anything else, should be placed on the wound to stop bleeding, nor should any irritating substance, such as kerosene, turpentine or stockholm tar, be applied.

If there is a foreign body, such as a stake, in the wound, it may be necessary to withdraw it to save further injury, otherwise it is preferable to leave it until the veterinarian arrives. If the stake must be removed, care should be taken not to break it off and leave a fragment deeply embedded in the tissues.

When bleeding has been arrested, it will be necessary to remove any dirt, clots of blood and other foreign matter very carefully. This may be done by gently syringing the part with normal saline solution (1 teaspoonful of salt to a pint of boiled water) which has been allowed to cool to blood heat, or with warm weak antiseptic, such as *Cetavlon* or *Dettol*, or soap solution. The hands should be kept away from the wound as much as possible and, if it is necessary to sponge the wound to remove foreign matter, use clean cotton cloth or cotton wool which has been soaked in the salt or weak antiseptic solution, and change the swabs frequently. Common ways of re-infecting a wound are by dirty hands and infected material such as tow and cotton wool.

It is advisable to clip the hair away from the edges of the wound with scissors. If necessary, as in the case of a suspected foreign body, the depth of the wound can be explored with a blunt instrument which has been boiled, or with the fingers after the hands have been thoroughly washed and scrubbed.

A human enema syringe is very useful in applying a continuous stream of a solution of salt or weak antiseptic to the wound.

Antiseptic solutions used are frequently too strong and have a detrimental effect on the healing of the wound.

In those cases where a hanging flap or large gaping wound makes stitching necessary, care should be taken not to pull the stitches too tightly and to make provision for drainage by leaving out the last one or two stitches on the lower side. Most wounds, especially punctured wounds, should not be sutured. Stitching of a wound is the finest way of keeping harmful germs in, or of introducing them if not already there, and the job should be left to a veterinarian.

Penetrating abdominal and thoracic wounds, and open joints, also require professional attention.

A fundamental principle underlying all wound treatment is to endeavour to provide suitable downward drainage for discharges from the wound. If such drainage is provided, most wounds tend to heal satisfactorily. Wounds which penetrate in an upward direction need little interference beyond ensuring that they remain open while healing from their deepest part and that they are reasonably clean on the surface.

Deep wounds penetrating downwards, and which form pockets, heal badly, as discharges collect within them and cannot get away. In the case of downward-penetrating wounds, it is necessary to use a knife judiciously in order to ensure that discharges can flow freely.

Wounds on parts of the body where there is a plentiful supply of blood, from which comes the repair materials, heal the best. Wounds in parts where there is a poor blood supply are slow to heal. Massage, hot packs, and the use of stimulating liniments around the wound encourage the blood supply.

When a wound persists in discharging and will not heal, it is a sign that infection, or a foreign body, such as a piece of wood, a splinter of bone or a piece of dead tissue is present. Such a wound should be opened right to the bottom, preferably by a veterinarian, and the offending material removed, or infection treated.

After an open wound has been thoroughly cleaned up in the manner indicated above, it will doubtless still be infected to some degree. Mild dry dressings, such as antibiotic dusting powders, should now be applied to the wound. These powder dressings are antiseptic and stimulate the formation of lymph, but are of most value in shallow wounds. With deeper wounds, such as a puncture of the foot, dusting powders may do harm by encouraging healing of the surface of the wound faster than the deeper tissue. For the latter type of wounds the injection of an antibiotic deep into the depth of the wound, will give the best results.

Systemic administration of antibiotics by intramuscular or sub-cutaneous injections and continued over a few days, is the modern method of controlling serious wound infection and is a routine procedure by veterinarians.

Punctured wounds are particularly liable to be contaminated deeply by tetanus spores and gas gangrene organisms, which find themselves in a favourable situation, namely with the absence of air, to multiply and elaborate their powerful toxins (see *Tetanus*).

The edges of a shallow wound may be encouraged to heal by painting with a solution of triple dyes, obtainable from any chemist, but the wound itself should be interfered with as little as possible.

Wounds open to the air, or only covered by a light protection, heal better than those heavily bandaged. It is sometimes necessary to use bandages to immobilize the injured area or to prevent further contamination or fly strike.

Where necessary, wounds may be protected to some extent from flies by smearing a fly-repellant dressing, such as 10 per cent citronella or dibutyl phthalate, around but not on the wound.

The application of stockholm tar is undesirable even around the wound; it is not a safe repellant; dust and dirt adhere to it, and it may retard healing of the wound. Should excess granulation tissue (proud flesh) occur, it may be checked by the application of 5 per cent bluestone solution (1 oz. bluestone to a pint of water).

It is again stressed that strong, irritating antiseptics should not be used in the treatment of wounds, as they only damage the tissues and lower the resistance of the wound to germ infection, and actually delay the healing process.

When the horse has sustained a severe wound, or suturing has been carried out, complete rest for two or three days will be necessary, but light exercise should be given as soon as possible as this is advantageous for good healing of the wound.

The majority of wounds will heal gradually by granulation under good nursing and a minimum of interference to the wound. However, serious complications, such as cellulitis, may occur as a result of virulent infection, and will require prompt treatment by a veterinarian. Shock is sometimes a complication of severe and extensive wounds, and will require professional treatment, as also will great loss of blood.

CONTUSED WOUNDS OR BRUISES

These are injuries to the deeper parts of the skin and the underlying tissues and commonly occur with only minor abrasions of the skin, although considerable swelling may occur from effusion of blood. They usually result from kicks from other horses, hitting an obstruction, or a fall. The importance of these bruises depends on the amount of damage to underlying tissue and on body location. A small contusion on a limb can be serious, owing to damage to the periosteum covering the bones, whereas a large bruise on the more fleshy parts of the body usually heals readily by resolution and absorption of the damaged tissue and blood which escapes from damaged vessels.

Treatment

Simple bruises, if treated early, respond very well to cold water applications with a hose. Alternatively, a pad of cotton wool or a cloth soaked in cold or ice water may be held over the bruise or applied with a bandage. The cold applications cause the blood vessels to contract and prevent further effusion of blood. This cold water treatment should be carried out for the first day, after which hot fomentations should be applied to the bruise and gentle massage given. Light exercise is beneficial. If the skin has been broken, the wound should be cleaned with salt solution or a very weak antiseptic and otherwise treated as an open wound. Serious contusions will require veterinary attention.

APPENDIX
COLOURS AND MARKINGS OF HORSES FOR IDENTIFICATION PURPOSES.

The following are the names of body colours and markings as approved by the British Royal College of Veterinary Surgeons in 1954, together with a few minor additions applicable in Australia.

BODY COLOURS

The principal colours are black, brown, bay, chestnut and grey. Where there is any doubt as to the colour, the muzzle and eyelids should be carefully examined for guidance.

Black: Where black pigment is general throughout the coat, limbs, mane and tail, with no pattern factor present other than white markings. Brown-black is also recognized.

Black-brown: Where the predominating colour is black, with muzzle, and sometimes flanks, brown or tan.

Brown: Where there is a mixture of black and brown pigment in the coat, with black limbs, mane and tail. Brown-bay is recognized.

Bay-brown: Where the predominating colour is brown, with muzzle bay, black limbs, mane and tail.

Bay: Bay varies considerably in shade from dull red approaching brown, to a yellowish colour approaching chestnut, but it can be distinguished from the chestnut by the fact that the bay has a black mane and tail and almost invariably has black on the limbs.

Chestnut: This colour consists of yellow-coloured hair in different degrees of intensity, which may be noted if thought desirable. A "true" chestnut has a chestnut mane and tail which may be lighter or darker than the body colour. Lighter coloured chestnuts may have flaxen manes and tails. There are various shades from light washy to deep liver. Limbs are never black.

Blue Dun: The body colour is a dilute black evenly distributed. The mane and tail are black. There may or may not be a dorsal band (list) and/or a withers stripe. The skin is black.

Yellow Dun: Where there is a diffuse yellow pigment in the hair. There may or may not be a dorsal band (list), withers stripe, and bars on the legs. The striping is usually associated with black pigment on the head and limbs. The skin is black.

Cream: The body coat is of a cream colour, with unpigmented skin. The iris is deficient in pigment and is often devoid of it, giving the eye a pinkish or bluish appearance.

Grey: Where the body coat is a varying mosaic of black and white hairs, with the skin black. With increasing age the coat grows lighter in colour. As there are many variations according to age and season, all of them should be described by the general term "grey". The flea-bitten grey may contain three colours or the two basic colours, and should be so described.

Roans: Roans are distinguished by the ground or body colours, all of which are permanent.

Blue Roan: Where the body colour is black or black-brown, with an admixture of white hair, which gives a blue tinge to the coat. On the limbs from the knees and hocks down the black hairs usually predominate; white markings may be encountered.

Bay or Red Roan: Where the body colour is bay or bay-brown with an admixture of white hairs which gives a reddish tinge to the coat. On the limbs from the knees and hocks down the black hairs usually predominate; white markings may be encountered.

Strawberry or Chestnut Roan: Where the body colour is chestnut with an admixture of white hairs.

Piebald: Where the body coat consists of large irregular patches of black and of white. The line of demarcation between the two colours is generally well defined.

Skewbald: Where the body coat consists of large irregular patches of white and of any definite colour except black. The line of demarcation between the colours is generally well defined.

Odd Coloured: Where the body coat consists of large irregular patches of more than two colours, which may merge into each other at the edges of the patches.

Note: The term "whole coloured" is used where there are no hairs of any other colour on the body, head or limbs.

MARKINGS

The variations in markings of horses are infinite and cannot be accurately described by a limited number of terms without certain arbitrary groupings. In some cases a combination of the terms given below must be employed. It is stressed again that all certificates of identification should, in conformity with later remarks, be accompanied by a diagram on which the markings are indicated accurately.

HEAD

Star: Any white mark on the forehead. Size, shape, intensity, position and coloured markings (if any) on the white to be specified. Should the marking in the region of the centre of the forehead consist of a few white hairs only it should be so described and not referred to as a star.

Stripe: Many terms have been used to describe the narrow white marking down the face, not wider than the flat anterior surface of the nasal bones, e.g. rase, race, rache, reach, streak, stripe, strip, etc.

The Sub-Committee recommend for the sake of uniformity that one term only be used and they select as being most useful for the purpose the term "stripe". In the majority of cases the star and stripe are continuous and should be described as "star and stripe conjoined"; where the stripe is separate and distinct from the star it should be described as "interrupted stripe"; where no star is present the point or origin of the stripe should be indicated. The termination of the stripe and any variation in breadth, direction and any markings on the white should be stated, e.g. "broad stripe", "narrow stripe", "inclined to left/right".

Blaze: A white marking covering almost the whole of the forehead between the eyes and extending beyond the width of the nasal bones and usually to the muzzle. Any variation in direction, termination and any markings on the white should be stated.

White Face: Where the white covers the forehead and front of the face, extending laterally towards the mouth. The extension may be unilateral or bilateral, in which cases it should be described accordingly.

Snip: An isolated white marking, independent of those already named, and situated between or in the region of the nostrils. Its size, position and intensity should be specified.

Lip Markings: Should be accurately described, whether embracing the whole or a portion of either lip. (See Flesh Marks.)

White Muzzle: Where the white embraces both lips and extends to the region of the nostrils.

Wall-eye: This term should be used exclusively where there is such a lack of pigment—whether partial or complete—in the iris, that it appears pinkish-white or bluish-white.

Showing the White of the Eye: Where some part of the sclera of the eye appears unpigmented (white).

Whorls: See Note 3.

BODY

Grey-Ticked: Where white hairs are sparsely distributed through the coat in any part of the body.

Flecked: Where small collections of white hairs occur distributed irregularly in any part of the body. The degrees of flecking may be described by the terms "heavily flecked", "lightly flecked".

Black Marks: This term should be used to describe small areas of black hairs among white or any other colour.

252

Spots: Where small, more or less circular, collections of hairs differing from the general body colour occur, distributed in various parts of the body. The position and colour of the spots must be stated.

Patch: This term should be used to describe any larger well-defined irregular area (not covered by previous definitions) of hairs differing from the general body colour. The colour, shape, position and extent should be described.

Zebra Marks: Where there is striping on the limbs, neck, withers or quarters.

Mane and Tail: The presence of differently coloured hairs in mane and tail should be specified.

Whorls: See Note 3.

LIMBS

Hoofs: Any variation in the colour of the hoofs should be noted.

White Markings on Limbs: It is recommended that any white markings on the limbs should be accurately defined and the extent precisely stated, e.g. "white to half pastern", "white to below the fetlock", etc. The use of such terms as "sock" and "stocking" should be discontinued.

GENERAL

Mixed: To be used to describe a white marking which contains varying amounts of hairs of the general body colour.

Bordered: To be used where any marking is circumscribed by a mixed border, e.g. "bordered star", "bordered stripe".

Flesh Marks: Patches where the pigment of the skin is absent should be described as "flesh marks".

NOTES

1. *Acquired Marks*: There are many adventitious marks (i.e. not congenital marks) which are permanent, e.g. saddle marks, bridle marks, collar marks, girth marks, and other harness marks, permanent bandage marks, firing and branding marks, scars, tattoo marks. Wherever these occur they should be described. If a horse should happen to be docked this fact should be mentioned.

2. *Congenital Abnormalities*: Any congenital marks or other abnormalities which cannot be included in the description under other headings should be clearly described in the certificate and indicated on the diagram where possible.

3. *Whorls, etc.*: The location of whorls or irregular setting of coat hairs should be precisely indicated on the diagram accompanying the certificate. Whorls should be shown by the use of a small circle with a central dot, indicating the centre of the whorl.

ROUTINE

The Sub-Committee recommended that the following order of certification should be adopted:

Colour, Breed, Sex, Age, Height; marks on head (including eyes) in the order described above; marks on the limbs, fore first, then hind, commencing from below; marks on body, including mane and tail; acquired marks, congenital abnormalities, whorls or any other features of note.

In Australia brands (if present) are always noted.

EXTRA TERMS

The following additional terms have been introduced with specific Breed Societies. They have been extracted from a paper presented at a conference of the New Zealand Thoroughbred and Standardbred Breeders Association, at Christchurch, N.Z. in June 1973 by Dr D. Zartmann of Albuquerque, New Mexico, U.S.A.

Breeds

(1) *Appaloosa*: Pattern, white patch over rump with spots in it or a leopard-like arrangement of spots. Sometimes carry a roan type of spotting.

(2) *Palomino*: A golden to light creamy body with white mane and tail.

(3) *The Paint or Pinto Horse*: Has a pattern with extensive white patches over a darker body colour. Varieties of pinto are piebald and skewbald.

Synonyms are paint, calico, and particoloured.

Two types of inheritance are *overo* and *tobiano* with characteristic spotting differences.

Overo is a pinto pattern with white patches which spread irregularly upward from the belly. The base colour is frequently roaned; mane and tail are usually dark. The legs are seldom white. The face is commonly bald (all white).

Tobiano is a pinto pattern with white patches which spread down from the back with borders which are usually clean-cut. Mane and tail may be white spotted or white and white legs are usual. The head is coloured but may have a blaze.

Colour Terms Only

Buckskin: A light yellowish coat with black legs, mane, and tail. Usually no black stripe.

254

Claybank: A type of dun but carries brown points instead of black.

Cremello (cream): Very pale diluted sorrel or yellow colour; may be nearly white and called pseudo-albino. Blue eyes.

Mouse: A mousy, diluted black. Basic tone is grey or yellow.

Seal Brown: Brownish black with traces of light areas on muzzle and flanks.

Sorrel: Light red or golden shades of body colour. Coat may be uniform in colour, or the legs, mane, and tail be lighter.

White: A true white is born white. Albino, in the technical sense, has never been documented in horses. Pure Albino is an animal that due to its genetic composition cannot transmit to any offspring a factor for pigment production. Apparently all so-called "Albino" horses have some pigment (dark eyes) or transmit a pigment factor to their offspring.

BIBLIOGRAPHY

REFERENCE BOOKS CONSULTED

F. ANDRIST, *Mares, Foals and Foaling*, J. A. Allen & Co., 6th impression 1962.

D. C. BLOOD and J. A. HENDERSON, *Veterinary Medicine*, Bailliere, Tindall & Cox, 3rd edition 1968.

J. F. BONE, E. J. CATCOTT, A. A. GABEL, L. E. JOHNSON and W. F. RILEY, Jr., editors *Equine Medicine and Surgery,* American Veterinary Publications, Inc., 1st edition 1963.

R. J. GARNER, *Veterinary Toxicology,* Bailliere, Tindall & Cox, 2nd edition 1961.

T. E. GIBSON, *Veterinary Anthelmintic Medication*, Commonwealth Agricultural Bureau, England, 1962

M. HORACE HAYES, *Veterinary Notes for Horse Owners*, revised by J. F. D. Tutt, Stanley Paul & Co. Ltd. 1965.

MERCK AND CO., INC., *The Merck Veterinary Manual*, Merck & Co., 3rd edition 1967.

W. C. MILLER and G. P. WEST, *Black's Veterinary Dictionary*, Adam and Charles Black, 6th edition 1962.

NEW ZEALAND DAIRY EXPORTER, *The Veterinary Handbook*, 1949.

NEW ZEALAND VETERINARY ASSOCIATION INC., Technical Committee, *Diseases of Domestic Animals in New Zealand*, Editorial Services Ltd., Wellington, 3rd edition 1971.

H. CAULTON REEKS, *Diseases of the Horse's Foot*, Bailliere, Tindall & Cox 1906.

F. H. S. ROBERTS, *Insects Affecting Livestock*, Angus and Robertson Ltd. 1952.

THE VETERINARY DEPARTMENT OF THE WAR OFFICE, LONDON, *Animal Management*, Her Majesty's Stationery Office, 1933.

UNITED STATES DEPARTMENT OF AGRICULTURE, *Diseases of the Horse*, 1942.

UNITED STATES DEPARTMENT OF AGRICULTURE, Yearbook of Agriculture, *Keeping Livestock Healthy,* Part 3, 1942

JOURNALS CONSULTED

Agricultural Gazette of New South Wales.
Australian Veterinary Journal.

INDEX

Abortion 1-2
Abscess 2-3, 13,
  bots and 17
  chronic 20
"Adult rickets" *see* Big Head
Age by the teeth *see* Dentition and
  ageing
Anaemia (haemorrhagic and haemo-
  lytic) 3-4
  see also Equine infectious anaemia
Aneurism verminous *see* Colic
Ankylosis 7, 171
Anthrax 4-5, 13, 36
  gastro-enteritis and 97
"Aphis disease" *see* Photosensitization
Apoplexy 133
Appetite "depraved" 5
  indigestion and 106-7
Arsenic poisoning *see* Poisoning min-
  eral
Azoturia 5-7
  lymphangitis and 123
  myositis and 6, 127

Back and loins 7
Bark-eating *see* Appetite "depraved"
Big Head (Osteomalacia) 8
"Bigleg" *see* Lymphangitis (sporadic)
Birdsville disease *see* Kimberley dis-
  ease
"Black water" *see* Azoturia
Bladder
  eversion of 8-9
  inflammation of (cystitis) 9-10
  retention of urine 10-11
Bleeding
  from nose (epistaxis) 12
  from veins 11
  accidental 12
Blistering 13
  inflamed kidneys and 112
Bloat *see* Colic, flatulent
Blood poisoning 13-14, 197, 198
  mastitis and 125
Blood pressure, high 11
Bloodworm *see* Redworm
Bone, inflammation of 14-15
Bots 15-19
Botryomycosis 20

Botulism (forage poisoning) 20
Bowels
  impaction of *see* Colic
  inflammation of (enteritis) 22-3, 97
  diarrhoea and 67-9
  displacement of 41, 97
Brain, inflammation and disease of 24
Bran mash, preparation of 24
Breeding *see* Parturition and Pregnancy
Broken-wind (pulmonary emphysema)
  24-5, 212
Bronchitis 26, 174
  drenching and 72
  laryngitis and 118
  see also Infectious equine bronchitis
Brushing 26-7
Burns 27-9
Bursitis 129

Calculi 29, 36, 41, 210
  see also Colic, obstruction (intes-
  tinal) Salivary Calculi and Urin-
  ary Calculi
Cancer 29-30
  of the eye 82
Canker 30
Capped elbow 31-2
Capped hock 32-3
Cataract 34
Catarrh (acute nasal) ("colds") 34-
  6, 118
  febrile respiratory *see* "Influenza"
  equine intestinal 107
Cellulitis 248
Cervicitis 235
Cheek stones *see* Salivary calculi
Chemical poisons 97
Choking 35-6
Cirrhosis of the liver 115
"Colds" *see* Catarrh
Colic 36-44, 163-4
  crib-biting and 48
  flatulent 39-41, 209
  impaction 10
  obstruction (intestinal) 41-3, 97
  pains 23

Colic—*continued*
  spasmodic 10, 33-9
  tympanitic *see* Colic, flatulent
  verminous aneurism 44
  watering and 237
  wheat engorgement 43
  wind *see* Colic, flatulent
  worms and 44
Colours and markings 250
Concussion, violent 193
Conjunctivitis *see* Eye
Constipation 41
  foals and 92
  hernia and 101-2
Contagious equine catarrh *see* Infectious equine bronchitis
Cording-up *see* Myositis
Corns 45-6
Coryza *see* Catarrh
Cracked heels 46-7
Crib-biting and wind-sucking 47-9
Cryptorchid horse *see* Rig
Curb 49-50
Cutaneous habronemiasis *see* Stomach worms
Cutting *see* Brushing
Cystitis *see* Bladder, inflammation of
Cysts *see* Tumours

Dentition and ageing 50-66
  permanent incisor tooth, parts of 51-2
  number of teeth 52
Dermatitis *see* Nettle rash, Mange, Leg mange, Lice, Queensland Itch, Photosensitization
"Dermoid cysts" *see* Eye
Destruction of a horse 67
Diarrhoea 67-8, 198, 214
  in foals 23, 68-9, 92
  hernia and 101-2
Digestive upsets
  bots and 17
  see also Colic
Dislocations 69-70
Displacement of the patella (stifle lameness) 70
Drenching horses 72-3, 131
  pneumonia and 156
Dyspepsia *see* Indigestion

Eczema 73-4
Emphysema 74-5
  see also Broken-wind

Encephalomyelitis—Viral 75-6
Enemas
  for constipated foals 92
Enteritis *see* Bowels, inflammation of
Entropion *see* Eyelids
Epistaxis *see* Bleeding from nose
Equine cutaneous papillomatosis *see* Warts
Equine infectious anaemia (swamp fever) 76-8
Equine viral arteritis (EVA) *see* "Virus abortion" and "Influenza", equine
Equine viral thinopneumonitis (EVR) *see* "Virus abortion" and "Influenza", equine
Exostosis 14, 15
Eye
  conjunctivitis 79
  "dermoid cysts" 84
  foreign bodies in 79-80
  habronemic conjunctivitis 82, 90
  keratitis 81-2
  periodic ophthalmia 83-4
  "swamp fever" and 76-7
  tumours 230
  see also Cataract
Eyelids
  cancer of 30, 230
  entropian 84-5
  inflamed 23

False quarter 85-6
Fetlock joint injury *see* Brushing
Fibroid swellings 20
Fistula 86
  of the poll *see* Poll evil and Fistulous withers
Fistulous withers and poll evil 2, 20, 86-9
  brucellosis in cattle and pigs and 87-8
Flies 89-90
Foal, rearing of orphan 91-2
Food rashes *see* Eczema
Forage poisoning *see* Botulism
Founder (laminitis) 11, 92-5, 195
  acute laminitis 94
  chronic laminitis 95
  metritis and 127
  superpurgation and 217
Fractures 95-6
  dislocations and 69-70

Frog 96-7, 227-8
  diseases of 96
  grease and 99
  see also Canker, Thrush

Gangrene, dry (Sitfast) 197
Gas formation 44
Gas gangrene *see* Blood poisoning
Gastritis *see* Stomach, inflammation of
Gastro-enteritis 97
Girth galls 98
Glanders 123
"Grapes" *see* Grease
"Gravel" *see* Urinary calculi
Grease, greasy heel 74, 99-100
"Greenstick" *see* Fractures

Habronemic conjunctivitis *see* Eye
Habronemic granuloma *see* Eye
Haematomas 2
Haemoglobinuria *see* Azoturia
Heart diseases 100
Heatstroke, heat exhaustion, sunstroke 24, 100
"Heaves" *see* Broken-wind
Heels, diseases of *see* Cracked heels, Grease
Hernia (rupture) 101-3, 175
  scrotal 102-3
  umbilical 101-2
  ventral 103
Hives *see* Nettle rash
Hock, diseases of 103, 208
  sprung hock 208
  thoroughpin 225
  see also Capped hock, Spavin Thoroughpin
Hoof, diseases of 104-6
  contracted heels 105
  brittle hooves 106
  see also Founder, Sidebones, Wounds
Hoofbound *see* Hoof, diseases of

Icterus *see* Jaundice
Indigestion (dyspepsia) 48, 106-7
"Influenza", equine 107-8
Infectious equine bronchitis 108-9
Infectious equine cough *see* Infectious equine bronchitis
Inflammation of udder *see* Mastitis
Inflammation of uterus *see* Metritis

"Itchy heel" *see* Leg mange

Jaundice (icterus) 109
  "swamp fever" and 77
"Jinked back" *see* Back and loins
Joint-ill (navel ill) 69, 109-11

Keratitis *see* Eye
Kidneys, inflammation of (nephritis) 112-14
  see also Colic
Kimberley disease or walkabout disease 114, 157
Knees, broken 111-12

Lameness 33, 47, 50, 99, 105, 115-17, 125, 191, 193, 195, 197, 198, 206, 207
Laminae, ("quick") sensitive 191, 192
Laminitis *see* Founder
Lampas (palatitis) 117-18
Laryngitis 34, 174, 118-19, 211
  drenching and 72
Lead poisoning
  roaring, whistling and 174
  see also Poisoning, mineral
"Leaking navel" *see* Pervious urachus
Leg mange ("itchy heel") 119-20
  see also Mange
Lice 120-3
Lungs, congestion of 11
Lymphangitis (sporadic) 123-5

Mange 125
  see also Leg mange
Mastitis (inflammation of the udder) 125
Melanoma 30, 126, 231
Melanosis 230-1
Metritis (inflammation of the uterus) 1, 126-7, 168
  founder and 94
  vaginitis and 235
"Monday morning sickness" *see* Azoturia, Lymphangitis
Myositis, acute (tying-up or cording up) 127-8
  azoturia and 6

Navel ill *see* Joint-ill
Navicular disease 128-30
Nephritis *see* Kidneys, inflammation of

261

Necrosis 86
Nettle rash (urticaria, hives) 130
Neurotomy 171
"Newmarket cough" *see* Infectious equine bronchitis
Nursing a sick horse 131-2

Ophthalmia *see* Eye
Osteomalacia *see* Big Head
Osteomyelitis 14
  tuberculosis and 230
Ostitis *see* Sore shins

Palatitis *see* Lampas
Paralysis 24, 132-3
Paralytic myoglobinuria *see* Azoturia
Parasites, internal 44, 97, 133-43
  anaemia and 3
  eczema and 73-4
  flies and 90
  see also Bots, Bloodworm, Redworm, Roundworm, Stomach worm, Pinworm, Tapeworm
Parturition 143-50
  premature 1
  natural presentation 145-6
  difficult 146
Periodic ophthalmia *see* Eye
Periostitis 151-2, 198-9
  see also Sore shins
Peritonitis 127, 152-3
  bots and 17
Pervious urachus ("leaking navel") 151
Petechial fever *see* Purpura haemorrhagica
Pharyngitis 34, 211
Photosensitization (trefoil dermatitis) 153-4
"Pica" *see* Appetite "depraved"
"Pink-eye" *see* "Influenza", equine
Pinworm 141-3
Pleurisy 154-6
Pneumonia 69, 127, 131, 156-7, 212
  founder and 94
Poisoning
  mineral 158-61
  plant 157-8
Poll evil 2, 20, 86-9
  see also Fistulous withers
Polyarthritis *see* Joint-ill
Polyps 161-2
  see also Tumours
Pregnancy 162-3

"Proppy gait" *see* Lameness
Pulmonary emphysema *see* Broken-wind
Pulse 219-20
Purpura haemorrhagica 163-4, 212
Pyaemia *see* Blood poisoning

Queensland Itch 164-6
Quidding 166-7, 218
Quittor 45, 167
  false quarter and 85

"Red water" *see* Azoturia
Redworm 18, 44, 133, 134-6
Respiration 220
Retention of afterbirth 167-8
Retention of urine 217
  see also Kidneys, inflammation of; Colic and Calculi
Rhinitis *see* Catarrh
Rig (cryptorchid horse) 169
  fertility and 169
Ringbone 15, 169, 195
  see also Sidebones
Ringworm 171-4
  man and 174
Roaring and whistling 174-5
  chronic 174-5
  strangles and 212
Roundworm 136-9
Rupture *see* Hernia

Saddle galls and sore backs 175, 197
  chafing and 175
  horse's condition and 184-5
  infection and 175, 178-9
  prevention of 176-85
  sitfast 175
  see also Girth galls
Saddling 175-84
  anatomy of horse and 175
  blood circulation and 180, 182, 184
  faults of 184
  injury and 176, 180, 182
  position of 177
  structure of saddle 182-4
Salivary calculi (cheek stones) 185
Sandcrack 185-8
  complete 186
Scirrhous cord 188-9
"Scours" *see* Diarrhoea
Seborrhoea *see* Grease
Seedy-toe 189
Septicaemia *see* Blood poisoning

Sesamoiditis 190
Shigellosis *see* Sleepy foal disease
Shoeing 188
   sandcrack and 188
   rules and 190-1
   sidebone and 197
Shoeing pricks 191-2
   swelling and 192
Shoulder lameness 192-3
   muscular atrophy ("sweeny") and 193
"Sickle hocks" 49
Sidebone 15, 169, 195-7
   draught horses and 195
   lameness 195-7
   partial 195-7
Sinus
   suppurating 45
   see also Poll evil
Sitfast 175, 197
   harness and 197
Skin diseases *see* Eczema, Mange, Nettle rash, Photosensitization, Queensland Itch, Ringworm
Sleepy foal disease (shigellosis) 197-8
Slipped stifle *see* Displacement of the patella
Sore backs *see* Saddle galls
Sore shins (periostitis, ostitis) 14, 15, 198
   see also Periostitis
Spavin 15
   bone 199-200, 202, 225
   bog 199, 202-3
Speedy-cut 203-4
   danger of 204
   splints and 204-8
Splints 15, 204-8
Sprains *see* Back and loins
Sprung hock *see* Hock, diseases of
Staggers ("megrims") 208-9
   ataxia and 209
Stifle lameness *see* Displacement of the patella
Stomach
   inflammation of (gastritis) 23, 97
   rupture of 209-10
Stomach tube *see* Drenching horses
Stomach worm (large and small) 139-41
Stomatitis 117
Stones in kidneys, ureters, bladder *see* Urinary calculi

Strangles ("distemper") 118, 174, 210
   as result of metastasis 211
   contagious disease 210, 212
   incubation period 211
   prevention of 213
Stringhalt 213-15
   Australian 215
"Summer sores" (Cutaneous habronemiasis) 90
   see also Stomach worms
Sunstroke *see* Heatstroke
Superpurgation 216-17
Suppression of urine 169, 217
Swamp cancer 90
Swamp fever *see* Equine infectious anaemia

Tapeworms 143
Teeth 166-7
   irregularities of molars 218-19
   see also Dentition and ageing
Temperature 219
Tendons, sprained 171, 192, 221-2
Tetanus ("lockjaw") 222-5, 247
   antitoxin 192
   incubation of 223
   prevention 225
Thoroughpin 225-7
Thrush 227-9
Tongue, inflammation of 229
   cancer of 229
   diet and 229
Toxaemia
   bots and 17
Trefoil dermatitis *see* Photosensitization
Tuberculosis 229-30
Tumours 24, 41, 210, 242
   in the nose 12
   botryomycotic 20
   benign 230
   see also Cancer
Twisted bowel 231-2
   strangulation and 231
   intussusception and 231
Tying-up *see* Myositis
Tympany *see* Gas formation

Udder, inflammation of *see* Mastitis
Ulcer 232
   bots and 17
Upper respiratory tract 118

Urinary calculi ("Stone" or "Gravel") 233-4

Urine suppression *see* Suppression of urine

Urine retention *see* Suppression of urine

Urticaria *see* Nettle rash

Urolithiasis *see* Urinary calculi

Uterus diseases of *see* Metritis

Vaginitis 235
   see also Metritis
"Virus abortion" 1

Walkabout disease *see* Kimberley disease

Warts (equine cutaneous papillomatosis) 236-7

"Water gripes" *see* Colic, spasmodic

Watering 237

Weaving 237-8

"Weed" 238
   see also Lymphangitis (sporadic) and "Monday morning disease"

Weights and measures 238-41

Wheat, engorgement with *see* Colic

Whistling *see* Roaring and whistling

Wind, broken *see* Broken-wind

Windgalls 242-3

Wind-sucking *see* Crib-biting

Withers, fistulous *see* Fistulous withers and Poll evil

Worm infestations *see* Parasites, internal

Wounds 243-9
  accidental bleeding 12
  classification of 244
  emphysema and 74-5
  peritonitis and 152
  shock and 248
  treatment of 245-8

"Yellows" *see* Jaundice